Neuromotor Immaturity in Children and Adults

Neuromotor Immaturity in Children and Adults

The INPP Screening Test for Clinicians and Health Practitioners

SALLY GODDARD BLYTHE

WILEY Blackwell

Library of Congress Cataloging-in-Publication Data

Goddard, Sally, 1957- author.
  Neuromotor immaturity in children and adults : the INPP screening test for clinicians and health practitioners / Sally Goddard Blythe.
    p.; cm.
  Includes bibliographical references and index.
  ISBN 978-1-118-73696-8 (pbk.)
  I. Title.
  [DNLM: 1. Developmental Disabilities-diagnosis.   2. Movement Disorders-diagnosis.   3. Adult.   4. Child.
5. Mental Disorders-etiology.   6. Movement Disorders-psychology. WL 390]
  RC451.4.M47
  616.85'88075-dc23
                                          2014000615

A catalogue record for this book is available from the British Library.

Cover image: Colorful gears forming a human brain together with one red big central cog. 3D rendering isolated on white.
© Adventtr / iStock
Cover design by Cyan Design

Set in 10/13pt ITC Legacy Serif by SPi Publisher Services, Pondicherry, India

1   2014

DEDICATION

For Peter Blythe

If I have seen further, it is by standing on the shoulders of giants
Sir Isaac Newton, Letter to Robert Hooke, 5 February 1675.

CONTENTS

4 INPP Screening Test for Signs of Neuromotor Immaturity in Adults 83

As a paediatrician with a special interest in neuro-development, I have been inspired by Sally Goddard Blythe's work and the work of INPP. To me, the link between balance and movement difficulties and learning difficulties is self-evident. Much, if not all, of what Sally Goddard Blythe has written in the past has been written for parents and teachers. Here is a book for doctors. Teachers and parents look to doctors for an explanation of their child's developmental problem, but doctors (particularly primary care doctors) consider neuro-development as 'specialist territory'. The doctors who have insight into child development work from child development centres, and these are often in specialist centres, which may not always be easy to access. However, children with neuromotor immaturity, whose development is not quite normal, and children with school-related problems are very common – so common that they could be considered part of the wider spectrum of normality. The medical culture now is the culture of specialism. The system demands that and parents expect a specialist opinion and a specific developmental diagnosis.

As a paediatrician with an interest in development, children were referred to me with a range of symptoms with the expectation of one or other specific diagnosis. Parents would often bring a checklist of symptoms for specific conditions (taken from a book or the Internet). Their child fulfilled most of the criteria. They wanted me to confirm their diagnosis, as it would then open doors to access funding from the education department. I was struck by the fact that checklists for separate specific conditions had so many overlapping symptoms. On examination, the physical findings overlapped considerably. Most had signs of neuromotor immaturity. I had this perception that most of these children were potentially normal children, who had for whatever reason, drifted from a normal developmental pathway, and with the correct support and nurture could be welcomed back to normal health and development.

Do all children have to be referred to a specialist? Should not a generalist have insights into common problems; into those conditions that are not yet diseases and disorders but deviations from normal; the grey areas?

A good health promotion and preventive service sees grey areas as its bread and butter! There was once a group of doctors who understood this grey area very well. These were the Community Medical Officers of yesteryear. They had wide-ranging community and public health roles including immunization and screening, and they were the school doctors. It was their role to identify children who may have learning difficulties in school. They knew their communities, their schools and teachers. They also knew their child development! They knew that there was a connection between subtle developmental difficulties and learning difficulties, and they also knew that soft neurology was important. They would follow up the children with developmental difficulties in school, and support their teachers, and be advocates for them if they needed additional resources. They would have welcomed this book because this book gives an understanding and an explanation of something they always knew. However, neurologists or hospital paediatricians were somewhat dismissive about 'soft neurology'. They were only interested in neurological signs which pointed to structural damage or specific neurological lesions. Immaturity did not interest them. The bodies that recommended the health and prevention programmes were either hospital (disease oriented) doctors or public health academics. Screening, they pronounced, had to be targeted to conditions with a medical label and medical intervention. Developmental surveillance was dropped from the programme.

Over the decades, the Community Medical Officers have been reorganized out of existence. Their duties have been divided up between health visitors, GPs, school nurses and community paediatricians. Community paediatricians' work is diluted between so many responsibilities (including child protection work, children in the care system, adoption and fostering and in working in specialist child development centres) meaning that the work for school is now confined to the statutory role of providing medical advice for the statement of special educational needs; this is an essentially bureaucratic role. They have little time left for that valuable preventive and health monitoring role that was the follow-up of children with developmental delays and motor immaturities and in liaison with the teachers.

We are told that various emotional and developmental disorders (e.g., dyslexia, dyspraxia, Asperger's syndrome, autism and ADHD) are on the increase, and we are facing an epidemic of mental health problems. Many mental health problems that society faces today have their origins in childhood. We cannot afford to drop our health promotion and prevention. We know that in general better nurture of our children could lead to better mental (and physical) health in adults, but beyond these vague generalizations, we have had no models or specific programmes. This book provides the evidence and the rationale and the methods for such a model.

Preventive health services understand the concept of monitoring the health of both individuals and populations. People don't need to be ill or unwell to qualify for health surveillance. We do need to understand what we are monitoring. We understand the concept of growth monitoring. The pattern of normal growth is well understood, deviations from the normal pattern are easily recognized and specific interventions and referral pathways have been worked out. In countries or communities where undernutrition is common, health care workers will give energy or protein supplements as soon as the child's growth begins to deviate from normal and long before the clinical signs of protein calorie malnutrition are evident. (The appearance of frank signs of protein calorie malnutrition in a child or a population would be considered a failure of the health care programme.)

Could we not apply a similar model to monitor development? Examining for neuromotor immaturity is more complex than measuring and monitoring growth. The issues are a little more difficult to grasp, the procedures a little less objective. The model is still the same. Neuromotor immaturity is common and can be identified before the criteria for specific disorders become apparent. Simple measures that can be incorporated into a pre-school or school curriculum and its benefits have been demonstrated. The measures used need not even be considered as interventions or treatments (any more than nutritional supplements are considered treatments). They are means by which the child can be encouraged back onto the natural pathway of health and normal development. Surely, this is not beyond the territory of a health service. Surely, it is relevant for primary care physicians to understand these issues and be able to examine and monitor children with these difficulties.

The curative model of health care (the model that likes the idea of specific diagnosis and specific treatment) is the model that the public and politicians buy into and is supported by the media and most of the medical profession. The medical profession likes certainty and is uncomfortable with grey areas – with 'soft neurology'. Our training and management system appears to steer us in the direction of a specific medical diagnosis and steer us away from grey areas. Yet, it is precisely the grey areas in life that lend themselves to proactive health care and primary prevention.

Relating behavioural difficulties and school-related problems (difficulties in reading, attention difficulties, dyslexia, etc.) to developmental issues may be a completely new territory to many non-specialist doctors. The first part of this book provides the research evidence and a neuro-developmental explanation as to why neurological immaturity in children results in subtle learning difficulties, and the difficulties these children have accessing the full curriculum.

The second part of the book develops the theme that neuromotor immaturity is not confined to childhood and reviews the evidence that many debilitating disorders in adult life (e.g., anxiety disorders, agoraphobia and panic attacks) not only have their origins in childhood but show clinical signs of immaturity in symptoms of movement balance and vestibular dysfunction, and as in childhood, these conditions can respond to remedial movement programmes. It is an exciting prospect that many of these debilitating conditions could be prevented by movement- and balance-oriented remedial education in childhood. All this strengthens the case for proactive programmes in childhood.

The clinical methods described in this book will enable the doctor to do more than take a history of development. It describes a thorough clinical examination to demonstrate motor immaturity signs in retained primitive reflexes. The link between these findings and the actual difficulties in the classroom can be explained to teachers and parents and an easily understood programme implemented. This is a fulfilling role for the doctor and empowering to parents and teachers.

I hope this book will be of interest to paediatricians (acute and community) as well as to primary care doctors. I hope it inspires school doctors. The section comparing the various schools of thinking in the tour and movement problems (sensory integration, Vojta, Bobath, INPP) will be particularly interesting to the school doctor. I myself have been aware of these systems and have referred children to various therapists practising these methods, but have not been quite sure of their precise differences in approach.

I hope it rekindles an interest in understanding neuro-development and in primary care developmental surveillance. Can we prevent this predicted epidemic of mental health problems in the future?

Dr Arthur Paynter
FRCP, FRCPCH, Retired Consultant Paediatrician
(Community Child Health)
May 2013

ACKNOWLEDGEMENTS

Peter Blythe, PhD, who amongst his many and diverse interests and innovations was the inspiration and originator of The INPP Method.

Dr Wolfgang Schneider-Rathert and Marian Giffhorn for suggesting the need for a screening test for clinicians to identify patients who would benefit from assessment and intervention using The INPP Method.

Dr Arthur Paynter for his contribution to the Foreword.

Thake Hansen-Lauff for her translation and corrections to an earlier manuscript which preceded this book.

Dr Editha Halfmann for her contribution to information about the Vojta Method.

Paul Stadler for information concerning Sensory Integration (SI) therapy.

Professor Peter Dangerfield and Dr Allison Hall for advice on medical terminology and relevance.

To children, parents, INPP staff and colleagues, who have shared pictures and given permission for photographs of test positions and examples to be published.

To the many children, parents, teachers, researchers and practitioners whose work in the past has contributed to the knowledge and methodology used today.

1
Identifying Signs of Neuromotor Immaturity in Children and Adults

If we ran a health service rather than a disease service it would focus on a physiological and evolutionary approach to health and education.

–Paynter, A. (2011)[1]

1.1 Introduction

Health and well-being are not simply the product of absence of disease. They are the sum total of a system and systems which function well together. *Dys*-ease as opposed to the pathological features associated with disease can result from lack of synergy within the functioning of systems. *Dys*-ease produces a variety of symptoms ranging from behavioural and specific learning difficulties in children to emotional and psychological problems in adults.

Problems arising from dys-ease or *dysfunction* can be compounded for social reasons by the operational restrictions imposed on the various professional disciplines responsible for identifying problems and prescribing effective remedies.

Parents are often caught in this professional no-man's-land, first seeking medical advice or reassurance when concerned about aspects of their child's development. If no underlying medical condition can be found, the family tends to be passed on to the next service in the system allocated to take on responsibility for the child's development. More often than not, this is education, but few educators are qualified to investigate or treat physical dysfunction, while health practitioners are not primarily concerned with educational difficulties. Spanning these two disciplines lies the domain of the educational psychologist, well qualified to assess and diagnose conditions in which physical dysfunction plays a part (e.g. developmental coordination disorder, attention deficit disorder, attention deficit hyperactivity disorder, ASD), but not in a position to provide a remedy for a range of physical symptoms. The result is that many of these children simply 'fall through the net' of services intended to identify children at risk and offer appropriate support or intervention – neither 'bad enough' for medical treatment nor 'good enough' – to realize their potential in the classroom.

This group of children is often subjected to numerous assessments, but go on to receive either inadequate or inappropriate intervention. Inappropriate intervention is the type that tends to

Neuromotor Immaturity in Children and Adults: The INPP Screening Test for Clinicians and Health Practitioners, First Edition. Sally Goddard Blythe.
© 2014 John Wiley & Sons, Ltd. Published 2014 by John Wiley & Sons, Ltd.

focus on the *symptoms* of underlying dysfunction instead of tackling underlying causes. If, for example, teaching more of the same does not ameliorate the presenting problem, while it can provide ongoing support, it is not the solution.

Similarly, a specific group of adults who present with symptoms which formerly would have been described as 'neuroses' may have a history of a cluster of underlying physical factors which have combined over time to make the individual more vulnerable to stress.

The now redundant term 'neurosis' describes relatively mild forms of mental illness that is not caused by organic disease, involving symptoms of stress (depression and anxiety). Neurosis affects only part of the personality, is accompanied by a less distorted perception of reality than in a psychosis, does not result in disturbance of the use of language and is accompanied by various physical, physiological and mental disturbances (as visceral symptoms, anxieties or phobias). The term neurosis was coined by the Scottish doctor William Cullen in 1769 to refer to 'disorders of sense and motion' caused by a 'general affection of the nervous system'. For him, it described various nervous disorders and symptoms that could not be explained physiologically. The term was re-defined by Carl Jung and Sigmund Freud over a century later, who used it to describe a variety of mental disorders in which emotional distress or unconscious conflict is expressed through various physical, physiological and mental disturbances, which may include physical symptoms (e.g. hysteria, hypochondria) or emotional symptoms (such as phobias, panic, anxiety and depression).

Today, many of these conditions do respond to medical and behavioural therapeutic interventions, others do not. In seeking to find a solution for those who do not respond to standard treatment or who are recidivists, further investigation for signs of neuromotor immaturity can help to identify additional underlying factors which may be involved in the continuation of symptoms and which might respond either to a physical intervention programme, combination of a physical programme and behavioural therapy or a different type of medical solution.

It is stressed that in all cases, this screening test should not be used to form a diagnosis but only as a basis for further investigations.

1.2 How to Use This Manual

The manual comprises four chapters.

Chapter 1 provides a general introduction for all readers. It includes a definition of Neuromotor Immaturity (NMI) and its implications and a literature review of links between NMI and specific learning difficulties followed by a description of the role of primitive reflexes in normal development.

The INPP method is described and compared with other well-known motor training programmes including Sensory Integration (SI), the Bobath therapy and the Vojta method.

Chapter 2 comprises the INPP screening test for use with children (4–16 years).

Chapter 3 explains the links between neuromotor immaturity and symptoms of anxiety, agoraphobia and panic disorder in adults.

Chapter 4 comprises the INPP screening test for use with adults.

Chapter 1 is recommended to all readers. Chapters 1 and 2 are relevant for professionals working with children; Chapters 1, 3 and 4 to professionals working specifically with adults. Professionals working with children and adults should read *all* chapters.

1.3 Overview

Neuromotor functioning provides one indication of maturity in the functioning of the central nervous system. It is also linked to functioning of the vestibular, proprioceptive and postural systems, which collectively provide a stable platform for centres involved in oculo-motor functioning and subsequently visual perception. Individuals with neuromotor immaturity frequently experience difficulties with related skills such as balance, coordination and visual perception, which can affect behaviour and educational performance in children and result in chronic anxiety and emotional sensitivity in adults.

Problems connected to neuromotor immaturity can be subtle and diffuse, failing to fit into any single diagnostic category but nevertheless undermining an individual's ability to function with competence and confidence. Children may present in a physician's consulting room as a behavioural problem or emerge in the classroom as a low achiever; adults seeking medical help may complain of a range of symptoms for which no abnormality is detected on clinical investigation.

One method of identifying signs of neuromotor immaturity is through the use of standard tests to assess retention of primitive reflexes and development of postural reactions and other tests for 'soft signs' of neurological dysfunction. Soft signs, which have previously been dismissed as being too generalized to be useful for diagnostic purposes, are minor neurological signs indicating non-specific cerebral dysfunction.

The presence or absence of primitive reflexes at key stages in development provides acknowledged signposts of maturity in the functioning of the central nervous system. Primitive reflexes emerge in utero, are present in the full-term neonate and are inhibited in the first six months of post-natal life as connections to higher cortical centres and frontal areas develop. Primitive reflexes are also suppressed in the course of normal development as postural reactions and muscle tone advance.

Primitive reflexes are retained under certain pathological conditions, such as cerebral palsy. In cerebral palsy, retention of the reflexes occurs as a result of damage to the brain or abnormal development which may have occurred pre-natally, at birth or post-natally (Bobath and Bobath,[2] Illingworth,[3] Capute and Accardo,[4] Fiorentino,[5] Levitt,[6] Brunnstrom[7]). Damage to the immature brain interferes with the normal process of maturation in a predictable, orderly, developmental sequence resulting in lack of inhibition, demonstrated by prolonged retention of the primitive undifferentiated patterns of movement control characteristic of infancy, accompanied by abnormal muscle tone, development of postural control, impaired patterns of movement and delayed motor development. Primitive reflexes also re-emerge in degenerative conditions such as multiple sclerosis and Alzheimer's disease, when demyelination results in deterioration of postural reactions and primitive reflexes are disinhibited. For many years, it was assumed that retention of primitive reflexes could not exist to a lesser degree in the absence of identified pathology, and therefore, primitive reflexes were not the subject of investigation in children with less severe motor delays or children who simply present with signs of a specific learning difficulty.

Physicians are familiar with the assessment of primitive reflexes as part of the paediatric neurological examination at birth and in the first six months of life, but if development is progressing normally at six months of age, these tests are rarely repeated in older children or adults, because it is assumed that primitive reflexes do not persist in the absence of pathology. This assumption has led to the development of a somewhat polarized view of how primitive reflexes are regarded within the medical professions; because there are no clear presenting symptoms of pathology, primitive reflex status in the older child is not assessed – a case of putting the telescope to the blind eye and saying, 'I see nothing through it'.

Children and adults who have *residual* primitive reflexes and/or under-developed postural reactions tend to 'slip through the net' of clinical services. Symptoms in the form of behavioural disorders, specific learning difficulties, under-achievement and anxiety states appear within the family, at school, in higher education and in the physician's consulting room, often in the form of 'secondary neuroses' or non-specific ailments, which have developed over several years and which are, in part, the result of increased levels of stress needed to recruit and maintain compensatory processes.

1.4 Relationship Between Neuromotor Immaturity and Learning Outcomes

Literature review

The concept that neurological dysfunction can underlie problems with learning is not new. Developmental disabilities were recognized in the nineteenth century chiefly as two forms of delay – cognitive delay in the case of mental retardation and motor delay in the case of cerebral palsy – but less severe symptoms involving discrepancy between intelligence and more specialized areas of language, learning, communication and social interaction including early infant autism only emerged in the twentieth century.

In the 1920s, the French were among the first to notice a link between 'motor awkwardness' and learning disabilities,[8] which they sometimes described as 'psychomotor syndromes'. In 1940, R.S. Paine described the presence of several isolated motor signs, such as awkwardness, tremor, hyper-reflexia or mild impairments in walking, in children with specific learning difficulties. He also pointed to problems in the perception of auditory or visual information, faulty concepts of space, diminished attention span, difficulty in abstract thinking and delays in academic achievement being characteristic features of children with learning disabilities. Mild epileptic symptoms were also noted as sometimes being present.[9]

In other countries, the term Minimal Brain Dysfunction (MBD) started to be used. MBD was formally defined in 1966 by Samuel Clements as a combination of average or above-average intelligence with certain mild to severe learning or behavioural disabilities characterizing deviant functioning of the central nervous system which could involve impairments in visual or auditory perception, conceptualization, language and memory and difficulty controlling attention, impulses and motor function,[10] but with more than 99 possible symptoms listed as diagnostic criteria for MBD by the 1970s, the term MBD was already being rejected as too broad.

Investigations into the presence of abnormal or immature reflexes in individuals with specific learning difficulties emerged from various schools of thought and disciplines in the 1970s.

In 1970, an Occupational Therapist (OT) at the University of Kansas carried out a study in which she compared the reflex levels of a group of neurologically impaired children with a group of children with no known neurological impairment. Every one of the group diagnosed with neurological impairment had abnormal reflexes. Eight out of nineteen subjects in the 'normal' or comparison group also showed some reflex abnormalities, and it was subsequently found that of these eight, one had behaviour problems and the remainder had either reading or writing difficulties.[11]

In 1972, Rider (OT), also at the University of Kansas, set out to assess the prevalence of abnormal reflex responses in normal second grade children comparing their results to a group of learning-disabled children. She found that the learning-disabled children had significantly more abnormal reflex responses than the normal children. Using the Wide Range Achievement Test (WRAT) scores as an independent measure, she compared WRAT scores on the basis of whether there were abnormal reflex responses or not. Children with integrated reflexes scored consistently higher on the achievement tests than those with abnormal reflexes.[12]

In 1976 at the University of Purdue, Miriam Bender examined the effect of just one reflex, the Symmetrical Tonic Neck Reflex (STNR) on education, and found that the STNR was present in 75% of a group of learning-disabled children but not present in *any* of a comparison group of children without a history of learning disabilities. She also developed a series of exercises designed to help inhibit the STNR and observed that as the STNR diminished many of the children's presenting symptoms improved.[13]

In 1978, A. Jean Ayres, the originator of Sensory Integration (SI) therapy, observed that one of the major symptoms manifested by children in disorders of postural and bilateral integration was 'poorly developed primitive postural reflexes, immature equilibrium reactions, poor ocular control and deficits in a variety of subtle parameters that are related to the fact that man is a bilateral and symmetrical being'.[14] One of the aims of sensory integration therapy was 'not to teach specific skills such as matching visual stimuli, learning to remember a sequence of sounds, differentiating one sound from another, drawing lines from one point to another, or even the basic academic material. Rather, the objective is to enhance the brain's ability to learn *how* to do these things'.[14] The objective was modification of the neurological dysfunction interfering with learning rather than attacking the symptoms of the dysfunction.

In 1994, Wilkinson carried out a replica study based on Rider's (1972) research. She found not only a link between residual primitive reflexes and specific learning difficulties but also identified a connection between residual primitive reflexes and educational under-achievement. Her findings indicated that one reflex – the Tonic Labyrinthine Reflex (TLR) – underpinned many of the presenting educational difficulties and that there was a relationship between the continued presence of the Moro reflex and specific problems with mathematics.[15]

Goddard Blythe and Hyland[16] investigated differences in the early development of 72 children diagnosed with specific learning difficulties compared to children with no evidence of specific learning difficulty using the INPP Developmental Screening Questionnaire.[17-19] They found significant differences in the developmental histories of the two groups with children in the specific learning difficulty group having a markedly higher incidence of early life events or signs of delay in motor and language development and factors related to the functioning of the immune system. Delays in learning to walk and talk were particularly significant in the group with specific learning difficulties.[16]

Other studies that have investigated the persistence of abnormal reflexes in children with specific reading difficulties have found the Asymmetrical Tonic Reflex (ATNR) to be present in children with reading difficulties[20-22] and a cluster of abnormal primitive and postural reflexes present in a sample of children diagnosed with dyslexia[23] and in children with attention deficit disorder.[24]

Investigations into the incidence of abnormal primitive reflexes in a sample of 672 children in seven mainstream schools in Northern Ireland between 2003 and 2004 revealed that 48% of children aged 5–6 years (P2) and 35% of children aged 8–9 years (P5) still had traces of primitive reflexes. Fifteen per cent[25] of P5 children had a reading age below their chronological age. Of these, 28 also had elevated levels of retained reflexes. Elevated levels of retained reflexes were correlated with poor educational achievement at baseline. In the younger group (P2), it was found that retained primitive reflexes correlated with poor cognitive development, poor balance and teacher assessment of poor concentration/coordination. Neurological scores and teacher assessment at baseline predicted poorer reading and literacy scores at the end of the study.[26]

Some research suggests that children growing up in areas of social disadvantage may also be at greater risk of educational under-achievement, not only as result of lack of appropriate stimulation in terms of opportunity for language development and reading, but also because of immature motor skills.[27]

Empirical findings also suggest that improvement in markers of neuromotor maturity (primitive reflex status) is associated with improvement in behavioural problems in some children.[28]

1.5 Neuromotor Immaturity in Adolescents

Adolescents and young adults can also be caught in the transition from compulsory education to establishing an independent adult life. Dr Lawrence Beuret, an MD practicing in Chicago, specialized in treating this age group, who start to experience problems for the first time in the final stages of secondary education or when they move into higher education:

Multiple factors converge in adolescents and adults with neurological dysfunction to create elusive and diffuse symptomology. Early reading and learning difficulties are generally absent; fine motor and writing problems are minimal; gross motor coordination is little affected; athletic ability may be above average and early behaviour is within age-appropriate norms. Academically 'not working up to potential' and emotionally or behaviorally not responding to accepted therapeutic or pharmacological interventions are the hallmarks of neuromotor immaturity in this population. This differs substantially from younger children whose symptoms closely correlate with the continued presence of primitive reflexes. The *under-development or absence of postural reflexes (reactions) has a much greater influence on symptom development in this older population.*[29]

Postural reactions and their role in supporting perceptual stability are described more fully in Chapter 3.*

Beuret went on to describe how the under-development of postural reactions has a much greater influence on symptom development and functional limitations in this older population, quoting De Quirós and Schrager[9] as providing one of the most detailed insights into the pathology created by incomplete development of this reflex system. In summary, he states:

Any deficiency in the critical systems of postural control must be compensated for by the intervention of the highest (most recently evolved) areas of the CNS. This follows the dictates of Jackson's Law – the most highly developed, most complex functions – will be sacrificed to maintain functions earlier evolved, more primitive, and more critical to survival. In humans these encompass high level and complex cortical activities such as comprehension, executive function, analytical, and synthetic abilities, as well as cognitive and processing competence.

In this older population vestibular-proprioceptive mismatch becomes the common thread throughout an individual's history, testing and treatment response. A history of motion sickness which continues beyond puberty or some abnormal responses to motion is present in all cases, although intensity and frequency is reported to be highly correlated with certain personality factors. Motion sickness – nausea, vertigo, headache and fatigue – being the most frequently reported symptoms, occurs uniformly in response to attempting to read or engage in some form of visual fixation (reading a map or using a screen) while riding in a moving vehicle. Other abnormal motion responses may be present concurrently with, or independently from, motion sickness. These can involve adverse reactions to lateral, vertical, interrupted and rotational forces such as those encountered on winding roads, hilly terrain, amusement rides, elevators and high speed trains.[29]

The hallmark of this group is that they have usually achieved high educational standards in the early stages of education through diligence and hard work, but either start to fail educationally or to develop emotional problems when the quantity of required reading increases, the academic environment requires a less teacher-directed approach, the demands to multi-task increase and, if entering higher education, both social and educational adaptations are required to achieve and integrate socially.

The INPP *screening* test is not sufficient to identify neuromotor immaturity as an underlying factor in this age group unless detailed attention is paid to tests for balance, soft signs of

---

*A more detailed description of neuro-motor immaturity in adolescents may be found in the chapter co-authored by Beuret in *Attention, Balance and Coordination – The A,B,C of Learning Success*.

neurological dysfunction and the developmental history of the individual. More detailed assessment for the presence of under-development postural reactions is usually needed with this age group.

1.6 Relevance of the INPP Screening Test to Health Practitioners

Family doctors and clinicians are in the front line of services available to identify signs of neuromotor immaturity in children, adolescents and adults and to make appropriate referral for further investigations and appropriate treatment.

1.7 What is the INPP Method?

The Institute for Neuro-physiological Psychology (INPP) was established in 1975 by psychologist Peter Blythe, PhD, with several aims in mind:

1. To research into the effects of immaturity in the functioning of the Central Nervous System (CNS) in children with specific learning difficulties or academic under-achievement and adults suffering from anxiety states, agoraphobia and panic disorder.
2. To develop reliable methods of assessing CNS maturity
3. To devise effective remedial intervention programmes

Children seen at INPP screening are examined on an individual basis using a series of standard medical tests to assess physical abilities:

- Gross muscle coordination and balance
- Patterns of motor development
- Cerebellar involvement
- Dysdiadochokinesia
- Aberrant primitive and postural reflexes
- Oculo-motor functioning (control of eye movements)
- Visual perception
- Visual Motor Integration (VMI)
- Audiometric examination and dichotic listening

The diagnostic assessment findings provide the basis for prescribing an individual regime of physical exercises which the patient carries out every day at home. Parents are responsible for supervising children's exercises each day. The exercises take between 5 and 10 minutes a day and are practised over a period of approximately 12 months. The patient's progress is reviewed at six to eight weekly intervals and the exercise programme adjusted accordingly.

INPP practitioners are professionals who already have the relevant professional qualifications to work in a field allied either to education, medicine or psychology and who have undertaken additional training in the use of the INPP diagnostic assessment and remedial intervention programme(s).

The INPP method is not intended to replace standard neurological examinations and psychological or educational assessments usually carried out by trained psychologists, remedial specialists and medical and other non-medical professionals. It does, however, provide a unique system with which to assess and remediate signs of neuromotor immaturity in children and adults for which no other cause has been found.

The following screening tests have been compiled to enable health practitioners to identify signs of neuromotor immaturity and provide the basis for appropriate referral. The screening tests should *not* be used in isolation to form a diagnosis.

Why assess posture and balance?

Posture is defined as the reflex anti-gravitational adaptation of a living body to the environment in which he lives. Posture depends on reflex acts which occur as a result of the integration of several sensory inputs and rapid adaptive motor reactions chiefly involving the visual, proprioceptive and vestibular systems. 'Posture means unconscious, inattentive, anti-gravitational adaptation to the environment'.[30] When reflex actions are functioning efficiently and at a developmentally appropriate level, they free 'higher' cognitive systems in the brain from conscious involvement in the maintenance of postural control. Conversely, if reflexes are not functioning in an age-appropriate fashion, conscious attention must be diverted to the adaptation and maintenance of postural control at the expense of attention to other cognitive tasks. Posture is also essential to support static balance, to provide a frame of reference for coordination and a stable platform for centres involved in the control of eye movements (oculo-motor functioning).

Why carry out assessments for balance?

Balance is a continuous dynamic process that describes the interplay between various forces, particularly gravity acting with the motor power of the skeletal muscles. A person has achieved equilibrium when it can maintain and control postures, positions and attitudes.[29] Balance is the end product of cooperation between proprioception, vestibular functioning, mechanoreceptors and vision, mediated by the cerebellum. Posture and balance together provide the bases for motor activities on which all physical aspects of learning depend:

> To have a sense of balance one has to know where one is in space at any particular moment. In vertebrates the point of reference for the balance mechanism is the head. The vestibular system (balance mechanism) informs the brain where the head is in relationship to the external environment. The proprioceptive system informs the brain where the head is in relation to the rest of the body thus informing it where the head is in relation to its supporting base. Any movement of any part of the body is made with reference to the brain's understanding of where it is in relationship to its structural support (base). With these three inputs the brain can instruct a model of the head and body in relationship to itself and the external world.[31]

Abnormal primitive reflexes in the school-aged child and adult provide evidence of lack of integration in the functioning of these three systems, which are fundamental to the sense of position and stability in space. Problems in control of balance can be manifested in a number of ways:

- Postural control
- Coordination
- Control of eye movements (affecting visual perception)
- Perception – for example, vertigo, sense of direction and disorientation
- Vegetative symptoms – for example, nausea, dizziness, palpitations and hyperventilation
- Psychological – anxiety and fear

Control of balance provides not only physical stability for moving in space but also acts as one of the main reference points for cognitive operations in space, including orientation (knowing your place in space, necessary to navigate through space), directional awareness (needed for way finding; understanding the orientation of symbols – for example, b and d, p and q and 2 and 5; being able to read an analogue clock or a compass) and mental operations in space involved in mathematics and the ability to visualize the motor actions needed for the ideation (motor planning) and execution of well-controlled movement.

What is the significance of static balance and dynamic balance to learning?

Static balance describes postural fixation, which consists of stabilized body attitudes. Static balance is necessary to be able to remain still in fixed positions. Children who have poor control of static balance often find it difficult to sit or remain still tending to be restless when engaged in pursuits which need to be performed from a fixed position, such as sitting at mealtimes, passive listening in class and writing. These children have a need to be 'in motion' in order to concentrate, and this restlessness can be seen as fidgeting and inattention. Paradoxically, the same children may have relatively good coordination when engaged in activities which involve action, such as on the sports field or in the playground.

Some research has pointed to a link between the ability to maintain balance while standing on one leg and specific language disorders.[32]

Dynamic balance describes the various translations and re-adaptations of postural role in performing efficient movements. Children with poorly developed control of dynamic balance will tend to shy away from robust physical activities, which involve translation of position in space – for example, carrying out forward rolls and vaulting over an object – consequently, they lack confidence in situations that require rapid adaptive reactions.

Adults tend to experience generalized feelings of insecurity which are thought to stem from lack of gravitational security; these include difficulties with orientation and way finding (particularly in unfamiliar environments) resulting in increased anxiety, which may later lead to avoidance. 'Secondary' psychological symptoms such as dislike or fear of new environments and desire to remain in familiar situations can be linked to problems with static or dynamic balance.

What is the significance of postural control to learning?

Posture is not only a neuro-*physiological* function that ensures physical stability and mobility against the pull of gravity, but it is also 'primarily a central neuro-*psychological* system which embraces a wide range of functional levels from spinal reflexes to higher mental processes'.[33] Postural control is linked to at least three perceptual systems – vestibular (balance), proprioceptive and visual – dysfunction in any one of these systems or how they operate together can affect the processes of perception on which all higher academic skills depend. Posture both supports and reflects the functional relationship between the brain and the body, to the extent that it has been said that 'there is nothing in the mind that cannot be seen in the posture'.[34]

What is the link between primitive reflexes, balance and postural control?

The Asymmetrical Tonic Neck Reflex (ATNR), Symmetrical Tonic Neck Reflex (STNR) and Tonic Labyrinthine Reflex (TLR), hereafter referred to collectively as *primitive tonic neck and labyrinthine reflexes*, both influence and reflect the functioning of the vestibular system and its interaction with other position and motion sensors.

1.8 How Does the Vestibular System Work?

The vestibular system or labyrinth comprises the non-acoustic elements of the inner ear and consists of three semi-circular canals and one utricle and one saccule located in each ear. The planes of the semi-circular canals lie approximately at right angles to each other. Each canal is filled with fluid (endolymph), which, as a result of its inertia, flows through the canal whenever the head experiences angular acceleration in the plane of that canal. Movement of the endolymph deflects the cupula, a structure which behaves like a critically dampened pendulum to seal an expanded portion of each canal called the ampulla. Information concerning the extent of deflection of the cupula is sent to vestibular receiving areas of the brain via sensory cells lying at its base. In addition to sending information about the rate of head movement, these signals also generate compensatory eye movements (nystagmus), whose main function is to maintain the stability of the visual world by stabilizing the visual image on the retina, despite movement of the head. The otolithic receptors in the utricle and the saccule act as multidirectional accelerometers. The main function of the otoliths is to indicate the head's orientation in relation to gravity, detecting information about tilt as well as linear displacement.

The vestibular system differs from the other five senses of touch, taste, hearing, smell and vision in that it has no special sensation of its own. We only become consciously aware of the vestibular system if its functioning becomes impaired or there is a disturbance in cooperation with other sensors involved in motion and position. This normally 'secretive' system then 'speaks' through the other senses, either heightening or dampening sensitivity, affecting levels of arousal and eliciting physical and mental symptoms of dizziness, disorientation and sometimes motion sickness.

Motion sickness has been described as the 'vestibular system's special form of sickness',[35] because motion sickness only occurs in the presence of a healthy and intact vestibular system, but motion sickness is in fact the product of conflict between information received by the vestibular system and other sensors involved in postural adaptation in response to different types of motion. Judging speed of motion provides one example of this – because speed is evaluated through two systems, by the vestibular system and the visual system. For the brain to accept the result, the two estimations must be coherent.[36]

Balance is the art of not falling; walking is a continuous sequential process of moving from stability through instability (while transferring weight from one foot to the other) and regaining stability; the ability to remain 'poised' between one phase of action and another depends on balance.

Berthoz described control of motor actions and thinking as a dual process in which posture and motor control are a preparation for action so that even our thoughts and dreams are an internalized simulation of action:[37]

> Our executive functions give us the capacity to inhibit cognitive strategies or innate reflexes that kick in too quickly. One might say to think is to inhibit and disinhibit; to create is to inhibit automatic or learned solutions; to act is to inhibit all the actions we do not take.[37]

Individuals still under the influence of primitive reflexes do not lack strength or power, rather they lack voluntary control over release of power and choice of actions. This can affect not only control of volitional movement and discrepancy between intended movement and performance but also cognitive processes. Berthoz goes on to say that 'inhibition enables competition, facilitating decision making, plasticity (flexibility) and consequently decision making and stability'.

1.9 Primitive Reflexes

The symmetrical tonic neck reflex, symmetrical tonic neck reflex, tonic labyrinthine reflex and Moro reflex.

Why have these four reflexes been selected for evaluation?

Reflexes that are connected to the functioning of the vestibular system have consistently been shown to act as barriers to learning and to play a part in the development of anxiety states:

1. The Asymmetrical Tonic Neck Reflex (ATNR)
2. The Symmetrical Tonic Neck Reflex (STNR)
3. The Tonic Labyrinthine Reflex (TLR)
4. The Moro reflex

The Asymmetrical Tonic Neck Reflex (ATNR)

The Asymmetrical Tonic Neck Reflex (ATNR) emerges in normal development at circa 18 weeks' gestation, at about the same time as the mother becomes aware of her baby's movements. Rotation of the head to one side elicits extension of the arm and leg on the side to which the head is turned and retraction of the opposite arm and leg. The ATNR increases in strength as pregnancy progresses and should be fully developed at birth in the full-term neonate.

In the first months of life, the ATNR plays a part in spontaneous movements, developing ipsilateral movements and acting as one of the earliest pre-conscious mechanisms for training hand–eye coordination (Figure 1.1). It is normally inhibited between four and six months of post-natal life (Figure 1.2).

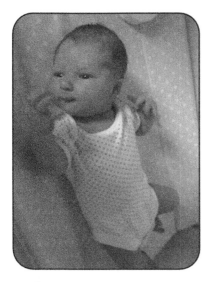

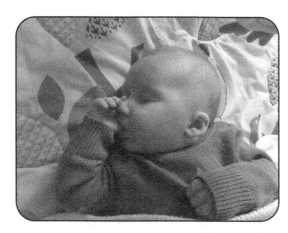

Figure 1.2 ATNR inhibited by the action of sucking in an infant at four months.

Figure 1.1 ATNR neonate.

Retention of the ATNR beyond six months of age can interfere with the development of subsequent motor abilities such as rolling over, commando-style crawling, control of upright balance when the head is turned to one side, the ability to cross the midline of the body when the head is turned to the affected side (potentially affecting bilateral integration), lateral eye movements and hand–eye coordination. Some observations have indicated a link between retention of the ATNR and failure to develop a preferred side of functioning.[38,39]

In the school-aged child, a residual ATNR can interfere with activities which involve crossing the midline especially writing position (Figure 1.3a), writing grip (Figure 1.3b) and control of the hand when writing. If it is present in combination with other reflexes connected to the control of the eye movements involved in reading, it can act as a barrier to reading. Prevalence of the ATNR has been found to be greater in some children with reading difficulties.[21] In adults, it can either affect control of balance and dependent functions when the head is turned to one side or be elicited as a result of postural or vestibular dysfunction.

(a)

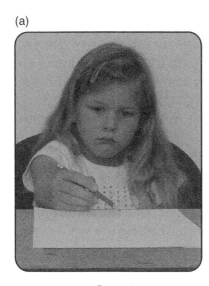

(b)

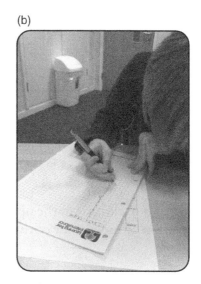

Figure 1.3a ATNR influencing writing position.　　**Figure 1.3b** ATNR influencing writing grip.

The Symmetrical Tonic Neck Reflex (STNR)

The Symmetrical Tonic Neck Reflex (STNR) is present for a few days at birth, recedes and then re-emerges between five and eight months at the time when the infant is learning to push up on to hands and knees from prone in preparation for crawling. The STNR should only remain active for a few weeks or retention can interfere with the next developmental stages of crawling on hands and knees,[†] sitting and standing posture and hand–eye coordination.

The STNR is elicited in a four-point kneeling (quadruped) position when head extension elicits an increase in extensor muscle tone in the arms and flexor tone in the hips and knees (Figure 1.4 and Figure 1.5).

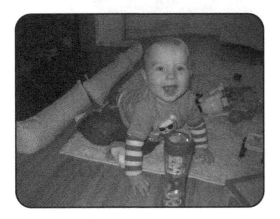

Figure 1.4 Symmetrical tonic neck reflex in extension.

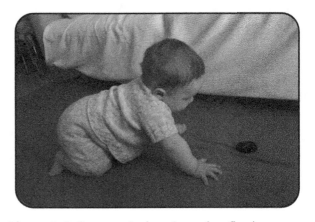

Figure 1.5 Symmetrical tonic neck reflex in extension.

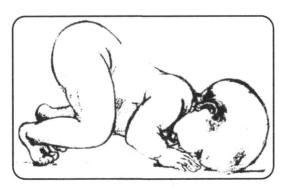

Figure 1.6 STNR in flexion. Reproduced with permission from Goddard SA (2002). *Reflexes, Learning and Behavior*. Fern Ridge Press, Eugene, OR. © Fern Ridge Press.

Conversely, flexion of the head elicits increase in flexor tone in the arms, causing the arms to bend, and increases extensor tone in the muscles of the hips and knees (Figure 1.6).

While the STNR has an important function in helping the infant to defy gravity, firstly in getting up on to hands and knees and secondly in helping him to pull to standing at the side of the cot, playpen or an item of furniture, it should not persist in the quadruped position after he becomes secure in the quadruped position or in the upright position once he has learned to stand unaided. If it fails to be suppressed by the time independent walking is established, distribution of muscle tone in the upper and lower halves the body can continue to be affected by head position or movement of the head through the mid-plane.

[†]Crawling on hands and knees is sometimes referred to as creeping, particularly in American literature on child development.

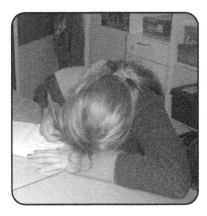

Figure 1.7 Sitting posture typical of an STNR in flexion.

In the school-aged child, this can be most readily observed in sitting posture when writing. When the child looks down at the writing surface, the arms want to be bend (and the legs extend), making the child lean further towards the writing surface, so that in some cases she may end up almost lying on the desk to write (Figure 1.7).

When the head is raised, the child is able sit up, but each time he or she looks down, the arms bend. If she extends her head, the opposite reaction occurs – the arms straighten and the legs bend. Children will try to find all sorts of different ways to get comfortable when sitting to write, including wrapping their feet around the legs of the chair or partially squatting on the chair (Figure 1.8, Figure 1.9, Figure 1.10 and Figure 1.11).

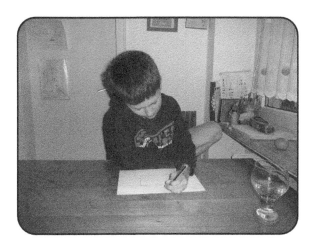

Figure 1.8 STNR influencing sitting posture.

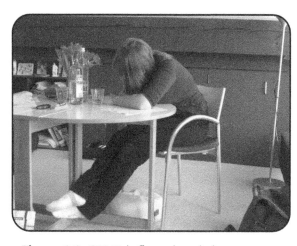

Figure 1.9 STNR influencing sitting posture.

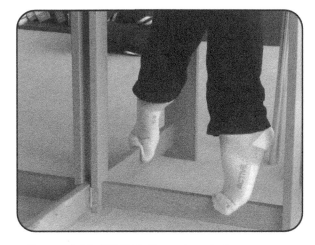

Figure 1.10 STNR influencing sitting posture.

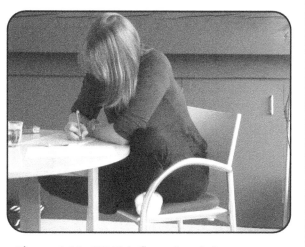

Figure 1.11 STNR influencing sitting posture.

In adults, the STNR can affect sitting posture (Figure 1.9, Figure 1.10 and Figure 1.11), upper and lower body integration, hand–eye coordination (particularly in the elderly) and visual perception.

In addition to making sitting awkward and uncomfortable, retention of the STNR in the school-aged child can affect specific hand–eye coordination skills including control involved in bringing the hand to the mouth when eating. Children with a residual STNR often have a history of being messy eaters finding it difficult to bring a fork, spoon or cup to the mouth without spilling some of the contents on the way. It can also interfere with the development of specific oculo-motor skills such as speed of accommodation needed to copy from the board or track an object approaching at speed (e.g. catching a ball) and the vertical tracking skills[40] needed to align columns correctly in maths and for judging heights.

The Tonic Labyrinthine Reflex (TLR)

The Tonic Labyrinthine Reflex (TLR) is present at birth and is a primitive reaction to gravity which recedes as head control, muscle tone and postural control develop. When the newborn is held in the supine position, if the head is lowered below the level of the spine, the arms and legs will extend (Figure 1.12).

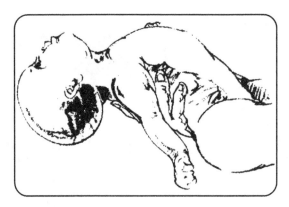

Figure 1.12 Tonic labyrinthine reflex in extension. Reproduced with permission from Goddard SA (2002). *Reflexes, Learning and Behavior*. Fern Ridge Press, Eugene, OR. © Fern Ridge Press.

If the head is elevated and flexed above the level of the spine, the arms and legs will flex (Figure 1.13).

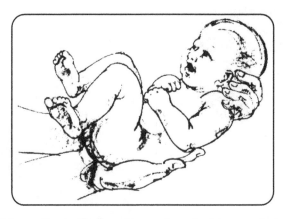

Figure 1.13 Tonic labyrinthine reflex in flexion. Reproduced with permission from Goddard SA (2002). *Reflexes, Learning and Behavior*. Fern Ridge Press, Eugene, OR. © Fern Ridge Press.

As head righting reflexes (postural reactions) develop in the first weeks and months after birth, the TLR is inhibited by higher brain centres and is replaced by a series of more advanced postural reactions, which facilitate adjustment of head position in response to movement of the body or the environment. These automatic head righting reactions provide the basis not only for control of balance and general coordination but also a stable postural platform for centres involved in the control of eye movements (fixation, convergence, accommodation and tracking) on which visual perception depends.

Retention of the TLR beyond three and a half years of age is associated with problems with balance, muscle tone and control of the eye movements needed for reading, writing, copying and mathematics and can also affect spatial skills. This is because spatial awareness and the ability to manoeuvre and carry out cognitive operations in space depend first on having a secure *physical* reference point in space.

Adults with evidence of a TLR usually experience generalized symptoms of insecurity linked to poor gravitational security and visual–perceptual problems.

The Moro reflex

The Moro reflex is present in the healthy full-term neonate and forms part of the routine paediatric assessment carried out shortly after birth. A weak or absent Moro reflex is seen in cases of upper motor neuron lesions; an asymmetrical Moro reflex at birth may indicate a fractured clavicle or Erb's palsy. It is inhibited at circa four months of post-natal life when it is gradually replaced by the adult startle or Strauss reflex.

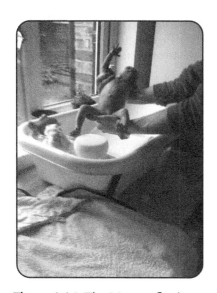

Figure 1.14 The Moro reflex in a neonate.

The Moro reflex is usually tested by placing the palm of the hand under the baby's head and lowering the head below the level of the spine. Unexpected vestibular stimulation such as rapidly lowering the whole body or striking the supporting surface will also activate the reflex. When the head is lowered, the arms abduct, the legs to a lesser degree; there is a rapid intake of breath; the neonate 'freezes' momentarily in the abducted position before the arms adduct; and the baby will usually start to cry (Figure 1.14).

Although the Moro reflex is most sensitive to vestibular stimulation in the first days of life, it can also be elicited by any sudden change of position or unexpected sensory event and is the only one of the primitive reflexes to have multi-sensory receptors.

Retention of the Moro reflex in an older individual is associated with a tendency to over-react and to be hyper-sensitive to specific stimuli. Although the accepted method for assessing the Moro reflex is rapid alteration of head position, the Moro reflex can continue to be elicited by other sensory stimuli at an older age if the specific sensory system involved is unable to filter or process sensory stimuli adequately. The reflex can also be elicited by destabilizing postural control if postural reactions are under-developed. Retention of the Moro reflex in older children and adults is associated with an over-reactive startle response and increased propensity to anxiety.[‡]

1.10 What Evidence is There that Intervention in the Form of Movement Programmes Aimed at the Level of Primitive Reflexes Improves Reflex Status and Educational Outcomes?

Traditionally, remediation of educational difficulties tends to be primarily aimed at treating the symptom, that is, focusing resources on teaching and practice of more reading, more writing, more spelling and more maths as is considered necessary. While this can be beneficial if the problem is a direct result of deficit in teaching or the learning of foundation skills, it will not ameliorate difficulties that arise as a result of defects in underlying physical skills that support higher aspects of learning.

The concept of using motor training programmes to improve learning is not new either. Kephart,[41] Frostig and Horne,[42] Getman et al.,[43] Cratty,[44] Barsch,[45] Ayres,[14] Belgau,[46] Kiphard and Schilling[47] and others all advocated and developed perceptual and developmental screening and training programmes to improve the perceptual–motor skills of young children to enhance learning outcomes. In 1975, Blythe and McGlown[17] developed the INPP programme for use with individual children aimed specifically at inhibiting primitive reflexes and stimulating the development of more mature postural reactions. A body of research into the effects of intervention programmes aimed at integrating primitive and postural reactions has gradually accumulated over the last 30 years beginning with small-scale independent studies, which have indicated, firstly, that primitive reflexes can and do respond to specific physical interventions and, secondly, that maturation in reflex status is accompanied by improvements in coordination and educational measures.[20,25,40,48–49]

In 1996, the INPP clinical programme was adapted for use in schools.[50] Research carried out on this programme has consistently shown that:

1. There is a significant decrease in active primitive reflexes and improvement in measures of balance and coordination in children who followed the programme compared to control and comparison groups.

[‡]A fuller description of all of the primitive and postural reflexes and their effects on functioning can be found in Goddard, SA (2002) *Reflexes, learning and behavior*. Fern Ridge Press, Eugene, OR and Goddard Blythe, SA (2009) *Attention, balance and coordination. The A,B,C of learning success*. Wiley-Blackwell, Chichester

2. There are improvements in drawing and reading in children who had both abnormal reflexes *and* who were performing below chronological age in these skills before introduction of the programme.[51–54]

3. Empirical evidence provided by reports from teachers and head teachers has indicated that there are improvements in behaviour,[55] particularly playground behaviour; children are quicker to settle at lessons following the exercises; and there are noticeable differences in children's poise and posture.

4. In one study carried out in Northumberland, five children had been referred to the Behavioural Support Service in the area. At the end of the first term on the programme, all of the children were removed from the support service's list despite the fact that no specific behavioural intervention had been given in the intervening time.[55]

5. A follow-up study carried out in Germany two years after a cohort of children had completed the school programme found that the participants had maintained the gains they had made two years after they had completed the programme.[56]

6. A study involving 139 children in four primary schools in Germany carried out between 2008 and 2011 indicated that children who took part in the INPP school programme showed greater improvement in measures of abnormal reflexes, learning outcomes and social behaviour compared to control groups who did not participate in the exercise programme. Children in a class receiving speech therapy made the most significant progress.[57]

1.11 What was Known About Exercises to Inhibit Primitive Reflexes? When was the INPP Method Developed? What has been Your Personal Experience Since then?

In 1969, when Peter Blythe, PhD, first became interested in the effect of aberrant reflexes on children with average to above average intelligence who had specific learning difficulties, there were no exercises available to directly inhibit the aberrant reflexes. Others, Berta and Karel Bobath, for example, had recognized the significance of aberrant reflexes when working with cerebral palsy but tried to teach children with cerebral palsy higher cortical movements in the hope the cortex could be trained to 'contain' the effect of the continued primitive reflexes.

Initially, Blythe and one of his students, David J. McGlown, developed specific movements designed to teach the CNS to inhibit the aberrant reflexes and stimulate the appropriate postural reflexes. Later, Blythe recognized that primitive and postural reflexes have a purpose – a genesis, a period of maturation and, in the case of the primitive reflexes, a limited period of function. When a reflex has fulfilled its purpose, it diminishes until entirely inhibited by the developing CNS. It was this realization which led to INPP's unique approach to reflex inhibition and integration.

The INPP clinical programme integrates reflexes in a number of different ways depending on the presenting profile of the patient. Some reflexes are stimulated; others are integrated by stimulating associated sensory systems; normal infant movements are replicated to help integrate reflexes; and in some cases, 'higher' postural reflexes are stimulated to assist in the inhibition and integration of developmentally earlier primitive reflexes. The INPP remedial programme is based on the results of the INPP neuro-developmental assessment and the developmental profile of the individual patient. In other words, the reflex status of the patient provides the basis for the type and developmental level of remedial movements or sensory stimulation recommended.

In 1996, the INPP developmental assessment and clinical programme was adapted by Goddard Blythe for use in schools.[50] This involved the selection of a small number of tests taken from the full INPP diagnostic assessment and adapted for use by teachers to identify children who have underlying difficulties with balance and coordination, evidence of three primitive reflexes and visual–perceptual problems, who would benefit from a daily exercise regime.

Goddard Blythe devised a general developmental movement programme to be used with whole classes of children or smaller selected groups. The programme was designed to be used under the supervision of a teacher who had attended one to two days' training in the use of the test battery and movement programme. The movements are carried out every school day for a minimum of one academic year, key elements of the programme being regularity (every day), repetition (using the same movements daily for several weeks) and duration (minimum of one year to complete the programme).

The exercises are based on movements made by normal developing infants in the first year of life. All children participating in the programme progress through the programme at the same pace, and teachers do not select specific exercises for individual children. The INPP programme for schools has been the subject of a number of studies.[58]

1.12 What is the Difference Between the INPP Method, Sensory Integration (SI), Vojta Therapy, Bobath Therapy and Others Working with Primitive Reflexes? What are the Criteria for Referral to a Particular Therapy?

The INPP method

The INPP method uses standard tests developed for use by medical practitioners to assess areas of functioning listed under Section 1.7. While the tests for gross muscle coordination and balance, dysdiadochokinesis, oculo-motor functioning, visual perception and laterality provide indications of the degree and specific areas of dysfunction, it is *the reflex profile* viewed in a developmental and hierarchical sequence which will provide the basis for remediation using a developmental movement programme tailored to the results of the individual assessment.

Exercises may be viewed in five functional categories:

1. Stimulation (primitive reflex) exercises.
2. Stimulation or training of the sensory system(s) that elicit the reflex, for example, vestibular training (other systems of intervention may also work in this way. For example, auditory training can help to reduce reactivity of a Moro reflex elicited primarily by auditory stimuli).
3. Use of normal developmental movement patterns which occur at the time that one or several reflexes are being integrated.
4. Stimulation of a developmentally later reflex to inhibit an earlier one.
5. Stimulation of postural reflexes.
6. Use of exercises devised to integrate on a particular reflex (constructed movements).

Remediation starts from the point of the earliest aberrant reflex and/or sensory system involved and works developmentally from the brainstem up towards the cortex. This approach led one student of the INPP method to describe it as 'Peter Blythe's "bottom up" approach to resolving specific learning difficulties'. While there are similarities in underlying theory with other diagnostic and remedial systems such as Sensory Integration (SI), the INPP method differs in its developmental approach to *stimulation–integration–inhibition*, using primitive and postural reflexes as markers of immaturity, indicators of level and type of remediation required and measures of progress during and after intervention.

Although the INPP method can be applied to children from as young as six years of age and in exceptional circumstances (brain injury or a history of severe neglect in infancy) to younger children, the INPP individual programme is most effective when used with children from seven years of age and upwards.

The screening test for use in schools is suitable for use with children from four years of age to identify signs of neuromotor immaturity, but children under six can find it difficult to perform the exercises slowly and precisely. For this reason, less specific movement programmes are more suitable for use with this younger age group.

Sensory Integration (SI) therapy

Sensory integration was developed by A. Jean Ayres, an occupational therapist who had originally studied at the Institutes for the Achievement of Human Potential in Philadelphia, an organization dedicated to the development of rehabilitation programmes following brain injury. SI is a therapeutic method primarily for treating individuals with learning and motor organization problems. The SI approach to learning disorders:

> does not teach specific skills such as matching visual stimuli, learning to remember a sequence of sounds, differentiating one sound from another, drawing lines from one point to another, or even the basic academic material. Rather the objective is to enhance the brain's ability to learn how to do these things.[14]

Although SI also involves the assessment of some primitive and postural reflexes, remedial intervention is provided through stimulation, training and controlling the input of different senses with the aim of eliciting more appropriate adaptive responses to sensory stimuli and improved organization in brain function. Therapy usually involves activities that provide tactile, proprioceptive and vestibular stimulation. The practice of SI as a therapy has evolved since A. Jean Ayres first developed it and presented it in her doctoral thesis. Some of the key principles and features of modern SI include:

- The assessment of the child's difficulties is vital in order to find out where the child's problems lie and how to plan treatment effectively.
- Child/therapist interaction (intensive).
- Child guided (often the child seeks out the sensory input he/she needs).
- Therapist aims to help the child to find this out for him-/herself and guides in the right direction so that he/she gets maximum benefit.
- Aims to raise the child's self-confidence.
- Does not aim to teach the child how to perform/carry out specific tasks but 'helps the child to learn', that is, by using the sensory systems to help the brain to organize itself.
- Uses play and different types of equipment.
- Helps the child to work out how to interact appropriately with their environment.

In recent years, there has been a dichotomy among different branches of practitioners of SI. While one school of thought now places primary emphasis on sensory factors with less focus on motor skills (a deviation from A. Jean Ayres' original ideas in which motor experience was an intrinsic part of sensory integration), another branch – Ayres Sensory Integration (ASI) – is at lengths to differentiate itself from the other SI therapies (brushing, weighted vests, weighted blankets, therapy ball chairs, etc.). ASI referred to the latter as sensory-based intervention in contrast to ASI where there is a strong emphasis on motor skills. The Ayres people refer to this in terms of praxis, action-projected sequences, bilateral coordination, and so on, as well as the tactile processing/sensitivities recognized by both groups as being a hallmark of sensory integration disorders. In this part of the dichotomy, there is great focus on the improvement of motor skills which would be in line with Ayres' original writing. The current trends are polarizing strongly in both the sensory-based intervention and ASI, each remaining steadfast to prove their validity in treatment.[59]

Vojta therapy

The Vojta method is well known in Germany and other European countries but is not used extensively in the United Kingdom. Whereas the Vojta method shares the assessment of reflexes, posture and movement capabilities with the INPP method, the Vojta method tends to be directed at rehabilitation of brain injury, for example, cerebral palsy, spina bifida, etc., and can be started almost immediately after birth if indications for therapy are present. Assessment and therapy are used primarily with infants and young children. Therapy concentrates on:

- Modifying abnormal reflex activity through the induction of a different neurological activity supplying to the patient a new corporal perception. Proprioception plays a key role in the process
- Improved control of breathing

- Fifteen to twenty minute sessions three to four times a day usually carried out by parents under the direction of the therapist

Therapy involves manipulation in addition to practising a range of developmental movements.

Theoretical basis to the Vojta method

The development of human movements from birth follows a hereditary and evolutionary plan starting from prone to the achievement of the erect posture and locomotion. Vojta described this as the principle of locomotion of postural ontogeny. Others have described this as ontogeny replicating phylogeny. Normally, motor activity is innate, and all children pass through similar milestones of motor development. The most important impulse for movement development is contact and interaction with the environment. The ability to react with posture is consistent with regular reactions of the body on voluntary and involuntary changes of position in space. Disturbance or impairment in the ability to react appropriately with posture affects the whole psycho-motoric development of the child, especially if it occurs during the first year of life.

The Vojta assessment uses a standard neurological test with additional tests.

The following criteria are assessed in relation to age (gestational age):

- Tone of the trunk and extremities.
- Holding and posture of the head.
- Antiflexion, retraction and opisthotonus of the head.
- Asymmetries.
- Quality of movement when flexing and extending the extremities.
- Supination and pronation of the hands and legs.
- Reaction of approach towards the surface.
- Primary reflexes including the crossed extensor reflex and the suprapubic reflex (pressing the symphysis, which is followed by stretching of the feet and legs). These two reflexes should be inhibited by the fourth month of life. Persistence will result in abnormal fixed movement patterns.
- Primary movements during the first year are also assessed, particularly rolling (supine to prone) and crawling, which are reflexive movement sequences controlled by the interaction of subcortical brain centres with the spinal level (cord).
- There are 10 different zones on the trunk, arms and legs from which the movement patterns are elicited. By applying varying degrees of pressure to different combinations of these areas, it is possible to initiate reflexive rolling and reflexive crawling.

Vojta states that in a persisting motor coordination disorder, it is not the automatic control of the postural reactions which is impaired but the central coordination of the different muscle groups (muscle flexing) which are crucial for motor development.

Indications for Vojta therapy:

- Irregularities of movement in infants
- Asymmetry of the chest
- Torsion of the neck

Table 1.1 Comparisons between the therapeutic approaches of SI, INPP, Vojta and Bobath

Differences	Sensory integration	INPP method	Vojta method	Bobath method
Therapy suitable for:	Children with learning and motor organization problems	Children with specific learning difficulties, neuromotor immaturity, under-achievement; adults with agoraphobia and panic disorder where visual–perceptual and vestibular dysfunctions are also present	Assessment of infants at birth, treatment of acquired neurological conditions and neuro-developmental problems	Acquired neurological conditions, children with neuro-developmental problems
Investigations: Therapist involvement:	Assessment Child/therapist intensive	Assessment Daily programme, 5–10 minutes per day, average duration 12 months Therapist contact at six to eight weekly intervals for re-assessment and adjustment of the programme	Assessment Therapist guided but carried out by parents under instruction from therapist Twenty minute sessions three to four times per day	Assessment Therapy sessions vary according to the needs of the patient
Type of therapy:	Child guided	Therapist-led programme carried out under parental supervision	Therapist led but also carried out by parents at home under therapist's direction	Therapist's active involvement in carrying out therapy sessions
Method of treatment:	Does not teach specific skills, entrains sensory systems and improved organization in functioning of the brain	Therapy aimed specifically at inhibiting and integrating primitive and postural reflexes to stabilize the foundations for balance, postural control, coordination, oculo-motor functioning and visual perception	Uses a combination of manipulation and pressure (deep proprioceptive stimulation) and movement to improve function	Treatment is tailored to clients' individual needs and is based upon an assessment of their abilities and analysis of their movement disorder. This is achieved through the use of specialized handling techniques that help to reduce spasticity and facilitate more normal movement

Brain level:	Remedial intervention tends to work from the cortex downwards	Remedial intervention uses movements that start from the brainstem and works up to the cortex		Remedial intervention may involve different levels of the brain but is aimed primarily at improving the ability of the motor cortex to control movement
Equipment:	Uses play and different types of equipment	Minimal equipment required		Uses specific handling techniques to help children to relax and mobilize their muscles and joints. This improves the child's quality of posture and movement, enabling them to move more freely and be more stable and comfortable
Professional qualification of therapist:	Occupational therapists with additional SI training	Therapists with professional qualifications in a field allied to medicine, education or psychology who have trained in the INPP method	Parent under direction of Vojta therapist guidance and instruction	Physiotherapists with additional training in the Bobath method

Vojta therapy is recommended following manual therapy for the treatment of Kinematic Imbalance due to Sub-occipital Strain (KISS) and should be continued until the child crawls:

- Palsy of the plexus: M. Erb
- Spina bifida
- Dysplasia of the hip joint
- Poor erection, low truncal tone, inversion or eversion of the feet, scoliosis, kyphosis, paraplegia, neuralgia of the lumbar region and the sciatic nerve and myopathy

Advantages of Vojta therapy

Its advantage includes a clear concept of assessment and therapy which can start from early in development (immediately after birth if applicable).

Disadvantages of Vojta therapy

The disadvantages include babies cry during treatment, mothers can find this distressing and fail to carry out therapy correctly and therapy becomes more difficult to administer between two and four years of age as the child resists being held in the required positions.

The therapy aims:

- Achievement of fluent bipedal locomotion
- Improvement of strength, coordination, muscle tone and function
- Improvement of several autonomic functions including breathing, swallowing, digestion, circulation, blood pressure, urination and bowel movement

There are seven indicators for Vojta therapy. If there are more than four abnormal indicators in relation to age/gestational age, therapy should be used; if there are more than five indicators, therapy should start immediately.

Even infants who appear to be normal can be affected and benefit from therapy. Examples of infants at risk are those who have undergone a difficult birth or required intervention at birth (CS, ventouse, forceps, Kristeller movement) or infants born with low tone and asymmetry of posture.

The best time to apply the method is the first year.

Bobath therapy

Bobath therapy was developed in the 1940s by Dr Karel and Mrs Berta Bobath. It specializes in the treatment of acquired neurological conditions such as strokes, head injury, multiple sclerosis, incomplete spinal cord injury and Parkinson's disease. It is also used to treat neuro-developmental conditions such as cerebral palsy and other allied conditions. It aims to improve the quality of life and optimize ability by encouraging and increasing movement capabilities and function.

It is primarily a way of observing, analysing and interpreting task performance using assessment of the patient's potential, which the Bobaths considered to be that task or those activities which could be performed by the person with a little help and therefore possible for that person to achieve independently where possible. The method also involves the use of various techniques. Bobath always advocated that the therapist should 'do what works the best' (Bobath, 1978).[60] In the present day, this means that while therapy is based on sound evidence when it is available, much of what therapists do has not been formally evaluated (Table 1.1).

1.13 What are the Top Five Medical Diagnoses Where Referral to INPP Should Routinely be Considered After Checking the Reflexes by Clinicians?

The INPP method does not claim to offer a 'cure' for any specific disorder. Rather, it aims to improve functioning and can be applied to a range of disorders. While the INPP programme has been used to assist in rehabilitation after brain injury, it was primarily designed for use with children and adults in whom dysfunction is evident, but no pathology has been identified. The diagnostic categories in which symptoms have consistently shown improvement following use of the INPP method include:

- Neuromotor immaturity
- Development Coordination Disorder (DCD)/dyspraxia
- Educational under-achievement
- Specific motor–perceptual symptoms associated with dyslexia
- Motor aspects of Attention Deficit Hyperactivity Disorder (ADHD)
- Motor–perceptual aspects of Asperger's disorder
- School phobia and selective mutism
- Agoraphobia and panic disorder when visual–perceptual and vestibular dysfunction are features of the presenting symptoms
  (Rehabilitation after acquired brain injury)

1.14 Screening Tests

The next section, which explains how to use the screening tests with children, has been compiled based upon evidence that has consistently shown that:

1. Maturity in the functioning of the central nervous system may be inferred from children's neuromotor skills.

2. There is a relationship between children's neuromotor skills and performance on motor dependent tasks.
3. Residual primitive reflexes respond to the INPP developmental exercise programme.
4. Improvement in neuromotor skills can have a positive influence on learning outcomes, emotional regulation and behaviour.

Factors assessed in the INPP screening test for health practitioners

- Balance
- Proprioception
- Primitive reflexes: ATNR, STNR, TLR and Moro reflex
- Dysdiadochokinesis

How to use the screening test

This test is for screening purposes only and should *not* be used to form a diagnosis.

It may be used to:

1. Identify children and adults with signs of neuromotor immaturity and related difficulties
2. Identify children and adults likely to benefit from the INPP reflex stimulation and inhibition programmes
3. Identify children who have issues related to neuromotor immaturity, visual–perceptual problems or auditory processing deficits who should be referred on for more specialized assessment, diagnosis and intervention

References

1 Paynter, A (2011) Personal communication.
2 a. Bobath, K and Bobath, B (1955) Tonic reflexes and righting reflexes in diagnosis and assessment of cerebral palsy. *Cerebral Palsy Review*, **16**(5): 3–10,26. b. Bobath, K (1980) *A neurophysiological basis for the treatment of cerebral palsy*. Blackwell Scientific Publications, Oxford.
3 Illingworth, RS (1962) *An introduction to developmental assessment in the first year*. National Spastics Society, William Heinemann (Medical Books Ltd), London.
4 Capute, AJ and Accardo, PJ (1991) Cerebral palsy. The spectrum of motor dysfunction. In: Capute, AJ and Accardo, PJ (eds), *Developmental disabilities in infancy and early childhood*. Paul Brookes Publishing Co., Baltimore, MD.
5 Fiorentino, MR (1981) *Reflex testing methods for evaluating C.N.S. development*. Charles C Thomas, Springfield, IL.
6 Levitt, S (1977) *Treatment of cerebral palsy and motor delay*. Blackwell Scientific Publications, Oxford.
7 Brunnstrom, S (1970) *Movement therapy in hemiplegia: a neuro-physiological approach*. Harper & Row, New York.
8 Dupre, E (1925) Debilite motrice. In: Dupre, E (ed.), *Pathologie de l'Imagination et de l'Emotivie*. Payot, Paris.
9 De Quirós, JL and Schrager, O (1979) *Neurophysiological fundamentals in learning disabilities*. Academic Therapy Publications, Novato, CA. pp. 146–147.

10   Clements, SD (1966) Task force one: minimal brain dysfunction in children. National Institute of Neurological Diseases and Blindness. Monograph No. 3. US Department of Health, Education and Welfare, Washington, DC.

11   Gustafsson, D (1970) A comparison of basic reflexes with the subtests of the Purdue perceptual-motor survey. Unpublished Master's thesis, University of Kansas.

12   Rider, B (1972) Relationship of postural reflexes to learning disabilities. *American Journal of Occupational Therapy*, **26**(5): 239–243.

13   Bender, ML (1976) *Bender-Purdue reflex test*. Academic Therapy Publications, San Rafael, CA.

14   Ayres, AJ (1973) *Sensory integration and learning disorders*. Western Psychological Services, Los Angeles, CA.

15   Wilkinson, G (1994) The relationship of primitive postural reflexes to learning difficulty and underachievement. Unpublished MEd thesis, University of Newcastle-upon-Tyne.

16   Goddard Blythe, SA and Hyland, D (1998) Screening for neurological dysfunction in the specific learning difficulty child. *The British Journal of Occupational Therapy*, **10**: 459–464.

17   Blythe, P and McGlown, DJ (1979) *An organic basis for neuroses and educational difficulties*. Insight Publications, Chester.

18   Goddard Blythe, SA (2008) *What babies and child really need*. Hawthorn Press, Stroud.

19   Goddard Blythe, SA (2009) *Attention, balance and coordination. The A,B,C of learning success*. Wiley-Blackwell, Chichester.

20   McPhillips, M, Hepper, PG and Mulhern G (2000) Effects of replicating primary-reflex movements on specific reading difficulties in children: a randomised, double-blind, controlled trial. *Lancet*, **355**: 537–541.

21   McPhillips, M and Sheehy, N (2004) Prevalence of persistent primary reflexes and motor problems in children with reading difficulties. *Dyslexia*, **10**(4): 316–338.

22   McPhillips, M and Jordan-Black, J-A (2007) Primary reflex persistence in children with reading difficulties (dyslexia): a cross-sectional study. *Neuropsychologia*, **45**: 748–754.

23   Goddard Blythe, SA (2001) Neurological dysfunction as a significant factor in children diagnosed with dyslexia. Published proceedings of the 5th International British Dyslexia Association Conference. University of York, York, April 2001.

24   Taylor, M, Hougton, S and Chapman, E (2004) Primitive reflexes and attention deficit disorder: developmental origins of classroom dysfunction. *International Journal of Special Education*, **19**: 1.

25   Bernhardsson, K and Davidson, K (1989) Ett Annorlundo sät att hjälpa med inlärningssvärigheter. The Educational Psychology Department, Gothenburg Education Authority, Sweden.

26   North Eastern Education and Library Board (NEELB). (2004) An evaluation of the pilot INPP movement programme in primary schools in the North Eastern Education and Library Board, Northern Ireland. Final Report: Brainbox Research Ltd. NEELB. www.neelb.org.uk. Accessed on January 15, 2014.

27   McPhillips, M and Jordan-Black, J-A (2007). The effect of social disadvantage on motor development in young children: a comparative study. *Journal of Child Psychology and Psychiatry*. **48**(12): 1214–1222.

28   Goddard Blythe, SA (2010) Neuro-motor immaturity as an indicator of developmental readiness for education. Paper presented at The Institute for Neuro-Physiological Psychology International Conference, Miami, FL. April 2010.

29   Beuret, LJ (2009) The effects of neuro-developmental delay in adults and adolescents. In: Goddard Blythe, SA (ed.), *Attention, balance and coordination – the A,B,C of learning success*. Wiley-Blackwell, Chichester.

30   King, LJ and Schrager, O (1999) A sensory cognitive approach to the assessment and remediation of developmental learning and behavioural disorders. Symposium sponsored by Continuing Education Programs of America, Illinois, March 1999.

31 Teale, M (2011) Explain how certain reflexes can affect control of balance. Essay submitted to The Institute for Neuro-Physiological Psychology. Chester, UK.

32 Schrager, OL and King, LJ (1999) A sensory cognitive approach to the assessment and remediation of developmental learning and behavioural disorders. A symposium sponsored by Continuing Education Programs of America, Atlanta, GA. March 1999.

33 Kohen-Raz, R (1996) *Learning disabilities and postural control*. Freund Publishing House, London.

34 Kohen-Raz, R (2002) Postural development and school readiness. Paper presented at the European Conference of Neuro-Developmental Delay in Children with Specific Learning Difficulties, Chester, UK, March 10, 2002.

35 Oosterveldt, WJ (1991) The development of the vestibular system. The 3rd European Conference of Neuro-Developmental Delay in Children with Specific Learning Difficulties, Chester, UK. March 1991.

36 Berthoz, A (2012) *Simplexity. Simplifying principles in a complex world*. Yale University Press, London.

37 Berthoz, A (2000) *The brain's sense of movement*. Harvard University Press, Cambridge, MA.

38 Gesell, A and Ames, LB (1947) The development of handedness. *Journal of Genetic Pyschology*, **70**: 155–175.

39 Telleus, C (1980) *En komarativ studie av neurologisk skillander hos born medoch utan Isoch skrivovarigheter*. Unpublished Master's Thesis. Gotherborg Univerisitet Pyschologisker Instruktionen, Göteborg.

40 Bein-Wierzibinski, W (2001) Persistent primitive reflexes in elementary school children. Effect on oculomotor and visual perception. Paper presented at The 13th European Conference of Neuro-developmental Delay in Children with Specific Learning Difficulties, Chester, UK, March 2001.

41 Kephart, NC (1960) *The slow learner in the classroom*. Charles E Merrill Books Inc., Columbus, OH.

42 Frostig, M and Horne, D (1964) *The Frostig program for the development of visual perception*. Follett, Chicago, IL.

43 Getman, G, Kane, E, Halgren, M and McKee, G (1964) *The physiology of readiness: an action program for the development of perception in children*. P.A.S.S., Minneapolis, MN.

44 Cratty, R (1973) *Teaching motor skills*. Prentice Hall, Engelwood Cliffs, NJ.

45 Barsch, R (1965) *A movigenic curriculum*. (Bulletin 25). Department of Instruction, Bureau for the Handicapped, Madison, WI.

46 Belgau, F (2010) *A life in balance. Discovery of a learning breakthrough*. Outskirts Press Incorporated, Denver, CO.

47 Kiphard, EJ and Schilling, F (1974) Body Coordination Test for Children (BCT). Beltz Test GmbH, Weinheim, West Germany.

48 Jordan-Black, J-A (2005) The effects of the primary movement programme on the academic performance of children attending ordinary primary school. *Journal of Research in Special Educational Needs*, **5**(3): 101–111.

49 Brown, CG (2010) Improving fine motor skills in young children: an intervention study. *Educational Psychology in Practice*, **26**(3): 269–278.

50 Goddard Blythe, SA (1996) *The INPP developmental test battery and developmental exercise programme for use in schools with children with special needs*. INPP Ltd., Restricted Publication, Chester.

51 Pettman, H (2001) *The effects of developmental exercise movements on children with persistent primary reflexes and reading difficulties: a controlled trial*. Mellor Primary School, Leicester. Final Report: Best Practice Research Scholarship Study. Department of Education and Skills.

52 Preedy, P, O'Donovon, C, Scott, J and Wolinski, R. 2000 *Exercises for learning*. A Beacon Project between Knowle CE Primary School and Kingsley Preparatory School. Department for Education, UK.

53 Micklethwaite, J (2004, December) A report of a study into the efficacy of the INPP School Programme at Swanwick Primary School, Derby. A controlled study of 90 children. Department for Education and Employment Best Practice Scholarship website. http://.teachernet.gov.uk. Accessed on January 16, 2014.

54 Hunter, P (2004) The effectiveness of a developmental programme designed to be used with children with special needs. MA Thesis, University of Middlesex, UK.

55 Marlee, R (2006) Personal communication.

56 Jändling, M (2003) The use of the INPP movement programme at a German primary school. Paper presented at the 15th European Conference of Neuro-Developmental Delay. Kiel-Oslo-Kiel, March 2003.

57 Giffhorn, M and Queißer, C (2012) Ruhe durch mehr BewegungKann sich die Schule selber helfen? Eine Studie über ein neurophysiologisches Übungsprogramm belegt positive Auswirkungen auf das Lernverhalten bei Schulkindern. Niedersächsisches Ärzeblatt. 12/12.

58 Goddard Blythe, SA (2005) Releasing educational potential through movement. A summary of individual studies carried out using the INPP test battery and developmental exercise programme for use in schools with children with special needs. *Child Care in Practice*, **11**(4): 415–432.

59 Stadler, P (May 2013) Personal communication.

60 Mayston, MJ (2001) The Bobath Concept Today. *Synapse*, Spring: 32–35.

2
Screening Test for Use with Children

The majority of tests in this section are suitable for children from 7½ years of age and upwards. Some of the tests may be selected for use with children from as young as four years of age, but users should follow the age guidelines if indicated at the beginning of each test.

2.1 General Instructions

Testing should be carried out with the child wearing loose clothing and in bare feet.

For timed tests (Romberg test and one-leg stand), a stopwatch with second hand should be used.

To ensure that the child has understood verbal instructions correctly, the tester should also demonstrate the first part of each test procedure.

Additional notes of observations made during tests should be recorded on the separate observation sheets provided and attached to the final score sheet.

Please note that certain tests are only developmentally appropriate from five or six years of age. Omit tests where it states that the developmental norm for the test is older than the age of the child being assessed, unless it states that the test may be used for *qualitative* purposes in a younger child. (Qualitative observations enable the tester to observe the quality of performance.)

2.2 Scoring

All tests are scored using a 5-point rating scale:

0. No Abnormality Detected (NAD)
1. 25% dysfunction
2. 50% dysfunction
3. 75% dysfunction
4. 100% dysfunction

Neuromotor Immaturity in Children and Adults: The INPP Screening Test for Clinicians and Health Practitioners, First Edition. Sally Goddard Blythe.
© 2014 John Wiley & Sons, Ltd. Published 2014 by John Wiley & Sons, Ltd.

2.3 Tests

1. The Romberg test
2. One-leg stand
3. Tandem walk (from seven years)
4. Fog walk (from seven years)
5. Thumb and finger opposition test (from five to six years)
6a. Quadruped test for the Asymmetrical Tonic Neck Reflex (ATNR) (from six years)
6b. Adapted Hoff–Schilder test for the Asymmetrical Tonic Neck Reflex (ATNR) (from seven years)
7. Quadruped test for the Symmetrical Tonic Neck Reflex (STNR)
8. Erect test for the Tonic Labyrinthine Reflex (TLR)
9. Standard test for the Moro reflex (adapted for use with older children and adults)

The Romberg test

The Romberg test was developed by German physician Moritz H. Romberg (1795–1873) to assess proprioception and control of static balance. The test is based on the premise that at least two of the three senses – proprioception (feedback received from the muscles, tendons and joints concerning body position), vestibular function (necessary to know one's head position in space) and vision (which can be used to monitor and adjust for changes in body position) – are needed to maintain balance while standing. The brain can obtain sufficient information to maintain balance if any two of the three systems are intact.

The Romberg test provides an indication of loss of the sense of position if the patient loses balance when standing erect, feet together and *the eyes closed*.

Above four years of age, a child should be able to stand in this position for up to 8 seconds without loss of balance and above six years of age 10 seconds, and adults should be able to maintain the position for 30 seconds. The patient may make two attempts to complete the required time.

The first stage of the test is carried out with the eyes open and demonstrates that at least two of the three sensory pathways are functioning well. The patient is then asked to close the eyes. If the proprioceptive and vestibular pathways are intact and functioning well, balance will be maintained. If proprioception is defective, as two of the sensory pathways needed to support balance are impaired or removed when the eyes are closed, the patient will sway and fall.

While a 'positive' Romberg sign is generally considered to be loss of balance on this test after the eyes have been closed, *qualitative* assessment of an individual's stability when standing in this position with the eyes open and closed can provide additional indications of problems in control of static balance and/or proprioception.

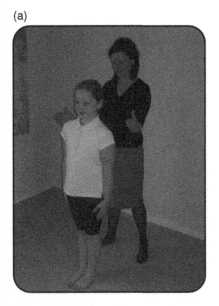

(a)

Figure 2.1a Romberg test (eyes open).

In children above the age of five to six years, the ability to perform the Romberg test has been considered an important milestone in postural maturation and links with another developmental marker, the suppression of synkinetic movements in the hands and fingers of the contralateral hand when the child is asked to carry out the thumb and finger opposition test.[1]

Test procedure: Romberg test

Test position

Standing up straight, feet together, arms and hands to the side, looking straight ahead (Figure 2.1a). Assessor should stand behind the test subject ready to catch in case there is a loss of balance.

(b)

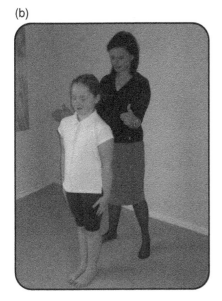

Figure 2.1b Romberg test (eyes closed).

Eyes open

The child is instructed to stand still and continue looking straight ahead.

This position should be maintained for approximately:

- 8 seconds (4 years)
- 10 seconds (6 years)
- 30 seconds+ (adults)

Eyes closed

He or she is then asked to maintain the position but to close the eyes and 'imagine' - pretend - that he/she is looking straight ahead. Hold the position for the age-appropriate number of seconds indicated earlier (Figure 2.1b).

Observations

Eyes open (qualitative observations)

- Is there noticeable sway?
- If so, in which direction – backwards, forwards, to the left or right side or in a circular movement?
- How much does he/she sway?
- Do one or both arms move out and away from the body?
- Does the face become contorted?
- Is there loss of balance?

Eyes closed

Note all of the aforementioned, paying particular attention to the degree of difficulty listed under 'observations'.

If the patient was able to maintain control of balance with the eyes open but loses control when the eyes are closed, the Romberg test is described as 'positive', indicating problems with proprioception.

If the test subject is able to maintain the position for the required time with the eyes open but balance is unstable and there is a marked increase in instability when the eyes are closed, this might indicate vestibular dysfunction.

If balance is impaired with the eyes open, there may be a problem with the cerebellum, but the Romberg test should not be used in isolation as an indicator of cerebellar involvement.

(Further investigations to ascertain whether vestibular or proprioceptive problems underlie difficulty in maintaining the position can be obtained during a more detailed diagnostic assessment asking the patient to perform the Romberg test first on a firm surface and then on a soft surface.)

The following conditions may also elicit a positive result on the Romberg test:

- Vitamin B_{12} deficiency
- Conditions affecting the dorsal columns of the spinal cord such as tabes dorsalis
- Conditions affecting the sensory nerves such as diabetic peripheral large-fibre neuropathy
- Friedreich's ataxia

Scoring for eyes open and eyes closed

0. None of the observations are noted.
1. Slight sway in any direction, slight movement of the arms away from the body and slight face or tongue involvement.
2. More marked sway, more marked movement of the arms away from the body and a more marked facial or tongue involvement.
3. Near loss of balance and need to extend the arms in a 'primary balance' position to maintain balance.
4. Loss of balance (positive Romberg test).

(Please note that a positive score is referred to as a positive Romberg sign. A score of 0 is referred to as a negative Romberg sign.)

One-leg stand or Unipedal Stance Test (UPST)

The timed unipedal stance test (also referred to as timed single limb stance, unipedal balance test, one-leg stance test and one-leg standing balance) is a simple test for measuring aspects of static balance and the ability to control one side of the body independently of the other (considered to be a precursor to the development of lateral preference.[2]) It can be used in a variety of settings and requires minimal equipment or training. It can also be used as one independent measure either during or following treatment to assess improvement.

Abnormal results on the Unipedal Stance Test (UPST) time with the eyes open are related to conditions such as peripheral neuropathy and intermittent claudication and are also linked to increased risk of falls (particularly in the elderly).

Precise developmental norms for this test vary according to the literature. Morioka et al. summarized the findings of several studies which showed that:

> Children will gain upright postural control equivalent to adults' when they are aged 7–10 years[3-6] or 9–12 years[7] according to various studies. The reason may be that children aged over six years can appropriately integrate the afferent sensory information required for posture control[8] and acquire the same upright postural control strategy as do adults.[3] Foudriat et al.[9] revealed that upright postural control in children up to three years of age is vision-dominant, but from that age onward, control will be gradually shifted to somatosensory-dominant control. Somatosensory-dominant postural control equivalent to that of adults will be achieved at ages over 6 years, which indicates that the development of standing balance may be nearly completed in the early school years. Morioka[10] has reported that the ability to maintain the one-leg standing position with the eyes open will dramatically improve in children within the period from late preschool age to early school age, and the improvement will slow down during late school age. That study indicated that the development of standing balance is nonlinear and that it is accelerated beginning at a certain age.[11]

Schrager[12] demonstrated that observations of both timing and body position while standing on one leg provide information about maturity of the central nervous system. He found significant differences in the performance of language-impaired individuals compared with a group with normal language ability on this test, surmising that the ability to control balance when standing on one leg and brain centres involved in language may be linked.[13] (He also noted that additional comparisons can be made between responses obtained on hard and soft surfaces with or without visual feedback.[12])

Test procedure for one-leg stand test (Unipedal Stance Test (UPST))

Test position

Instruct the child to stand on one leg and to 'maintain this position as long as you can'. Time (in seconds) the length of time the child can maintain the position without loss of balance, or placing the other foot on the ground. Repeat the procedure using the other foot.

Using a stopwatch, time how many seconds the subject is able to maintain balance while standing on one leg without moving the position of the foot on which he/she is standing. (Observe the test subject not the stopwatch.)

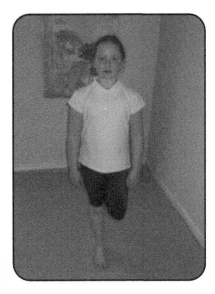

Figure 2.2 Test position for the one-leg stand.

Time commences when the subject raises the foot off the floor. Time ends when the subject either:

- Uses the arms, for example, extends them
- Uses the raised foot (moves it towards or away from the standing limb or touches the floor)
- Moves the weight-bearing foot to maintain his/her balance (Figure 2.2)

Developmental norms

Developmental norms for this test vary between different sources. Some sources state 15 seconds at six years of age and 20 seconds at seven years of age.[14] Others list the scale shown in the following:

3 years	2 seconds
4 years	4–8 seconds
5 years	8 seconds using left or right foot
6 years	20 seconds using left or right foot
8 years+	30 seconds using left or right foot

Observations

Inability to stand on one leg for the age-appropriate number of seconds may suggest underlying vestibular/postural immaturity in presenting difficulties.

Also note any marked compensatory or 'overflow' movements of the arms, opposite leg, mouth or hands when carrying out this test.

Scoring

Score for how many seconds the subject is able to maintain balance on one leg for left *and* right legs:

0. No abnormality detected
1. Two seconds less than normal time in seconds for age of child
2. Four seconds less than normal time in seconds for age of child
3. Six seconds less than normal time for age of child
4. Eight seconds or more less than normal time for age of child

Tests for 'soft signs' of neurological dysfunction: The Tandem and Fog walks

The Tandem and Fog walks are tests for 'soft signs' of neurological dysfunction. Neurological Soft Signs (NSS) are minor ('soft') neurological abnormalities in sensory and motor performance identified by clinical examination. There is still a lack of consensus on the neuro-dysfunctional area underlying NSS; some authors suggest that NSS reflect a failure in the integration within or between sensory and motor systems,[15] whereas others advocate deficits in neuronal circuits involving subcortical structures (e.g. basal ganglia, brainstem and limbic system).[16] While NSS do not identify aetiology, they can provide useful markers of possible CNS involvement in presenting symptoms and additional tools with which to evaluate change during or following intervention.

High soft sign scores have been shown to be related to significantly worse performance on measures of cognition, coordination and behaviour in mainstream school children.[17]

The Tandem walk

The Tandem walk is suitable for use with children *from seven* years of age.[18]

It is a test used primarily to assess balance, gait and signs of possible cerebellar involvement.

Patients with *truncal ataxia* caused by damage to the cerebellar vermis or associated pathways will have particular difficulty with this task, since they tend to have a wide-based, unsteady gait and become more unsteady when attempting to keep their feet close together.

Children with neurological immaturity will tend to show signs of clumsiness, accessory movements and loss of control of balance and coordination on this test. The Tandem walk can also reveal difficulty with control of balance and postural adjustment at the midline and proprioception. Evidence of poor proprioceptive awareness may be observed in accuracy of foot placement when carrying out the test.

(a)

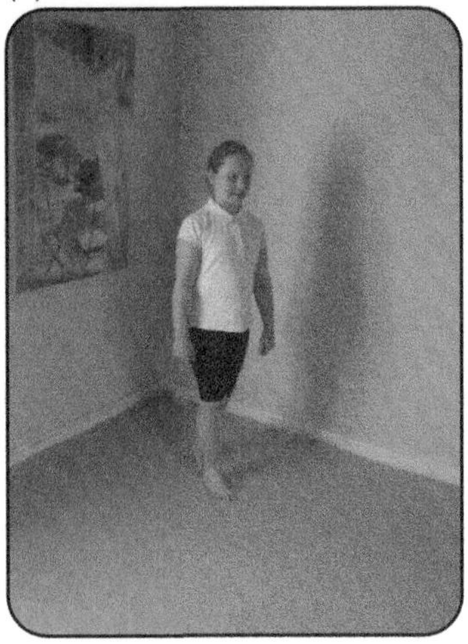

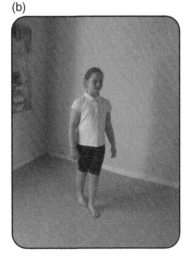

Figure 2.3a Tandem walk forwards.

(b)

Figure 2.3b Tandem walk backwards.

Both the Tandem walk and walking on the outsides of the feet (Fog walk) are carried out first forwards and then backwards. When going forwards, the primary sensory system involved in coordination is vision; when going backwards, balance and proprioception take over the leading roles. If a child's performance is *consistently and significantly* better on *both* tests in one direction only, it might indicate:

1. Forwards better than backwards – vision is being used to compensate for difficulties with balance and/or proprioception.
2. Backwards better than forwards – there may be a problem with vision or vision is not well calibrated with balance and proprioception.

(When applying this test to children or adolescents who have either recently undergone or are undergoing a rapid growth spurt, balance and/or accuracy of foot placement may be temporarily impaired. If it is suspected that growth is a factor in undermining balance and coordination, the test should be repeated one month later.)

Test procedure: The Tandem walk

Test position: standing and eyes open

Instruct the child to walk *slowly* in a straight line with the heel of the leading foot making contact with the toes of the trailing foot each time the leading foot is placed on the ground (Figure 2.3a and Figure 2.3b):

1. Forwards (Figure 2.3a)
2. Backwards (Figure 2.3b) (toe of the leading foot making contact with heel of the trailing foot when the leading foot is placed on the ground)

Score separately for forwards and backwards.

Observations

General: Note any problems with balance, coordination and position of the limbs.

- Observe control of balance. Is there marked difficulty in maintaining balance?
- Does the child need to hold his/her arms out in a primary balance position or use excessive arm movements in order to carry out the test (indicative of difficulty with maintaining balance over a narrow base of support)?
- Check accuracy of foot placement (proprioceptive awareness).
- Note degree of difficulty/concentration used to carry out the task.
- Note any 'overflow' of movement, for example, facial, mouth, tongue or hand involvement.
- Note the speed at which the test is performed. If too fast, remind the child once to slow down. If the child can maintain control only when moving fast and any of the aforementioned signs emerge when movement is slowed down, it might indicate that the child uses momentum to compensate for poor control of balance. (This is particularly prevalent in children who find it difficult to remain still.)

Scoring

0. NAD
1. Minimal problems noted with the following: Balance or foot placement, tendency to fixate visually on one point, slight facial involvement, tendency to look down and slight hand or arm involvement
2. Increase in any or several of the aforementioned observations, use of 'primary balance' position, some difficulty in controlling balance at the midline and test performed too fast
3. Near loss of balance, arms extended, sway in arms or body and inaccuracy in foot placement
4. Loss of balance with or without marked increase in any of the aforementioned observations

The Fog walk (1963[19]) (walking on the outsides of the feet)

The Fog walk is a test used in medicine to elicit vertical synkinesia.

The child is instructed to walk slowly in a straight line for a distance of 3–4 m on the outsides of the feet keeping the arms to the sides.

Going on to the outsides of the feet can elicit abnormal posturing of the upper extremities. Associated movements should disappear by 10–13 years of age, but the test may be used *qualitatively* with younger children from 7½ years of age.[20]

Associated movements are defined as movements that accompany a motor function, are not involved in the specific motor function and are not necessary to its performance. The persistence of associated movements is a sign supporting other evidence of immaturity in the brain or of poor development of discriminatory, selective motor activity.[19]

(a)

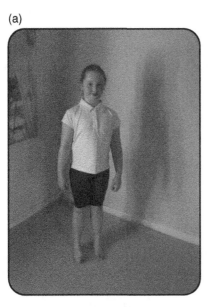

Figure 2.4a Starting position for the Fog walk.

Test procedure: The Fog walk

Test position: standing and eyes open

Instruct the child to go on to the outsides of the feet and then walk *slowly* in a straight line for a distance of approximately 4 m (Figure 2.4a):

1. Forwards
2. Backwards

After completing the distance forwards, instruct the child to stop, put the feet together and stand still and then to repeat the procedure going backwards. Score separately for forwards and backwards.

Observations

- Note any difficulty staying on the outside of the feet (e.g. tendency to walk on the heels).
- Alteration in posture and/or gait (Figure 2.4b) from mild to simian posture or gait.
- Coordination.
- Position of the hands and arms such as partial rotation and/or gripping in one or both hands, hemiplegia.
- Involuntary involvement or movements of the mouth.

(b)

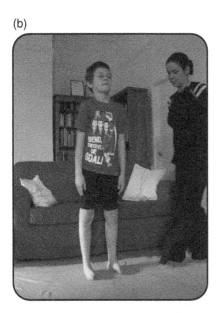

Figure 2.4b Vertical synkinesia evident when assuming the start position for the Fog walk.

Note that the test subject shown in Figure 2.4a does exhibit a slight positive score (1) in the hand position and posture when she assumes the start position for the test. More marked signs of vertical synkinesia and facial involvement are evident in the older child shown in Figure 2.4b.

Scoring

  0. NAD
  1. Slight involuntary hand involvement on one side
  2. Hand involvement on both sides and/or slight postural alteration or not fully on the outsides of the feet and/or facial involvement
  3. Simian posture or stiff gait with homolateral movements or marked hemiplegia
  4. Marked simian posture and unable to move or complete the task

Finger and thumb opposition test

By 38 months of age, a child should be able to oppose the thumb to each of the four fingers of the same hand in succession.[21,22] This ability improves between three and eight years of age, although some mirroring of movement may still be observed up to 10 years of age.[23] Difficulty in touching the thumb with the fingers of the same hand in systematic succession may be indicative of minor cerebellar dysfunction. Satz et al.[24] demonstrated that difficulty with thumb and finger opposition was among one of the strongest predictors of learning disabilities in the first years of primary (elementary) school.

Qualitative assessment using this test is suitable for use with children from 5½ to 6 years of age. Difficulties with thumb and finger opposition can contribute to difficulty with handwriting and are often found in children with a history of delayed speech.

The ability to suppress synergetic (mirroring movements on the opposite side of the body) improves rapidly between the ages of five and seven years and reflects the ability to act independently with each side of the body, which is considered to be a necessary starting point for laterality.[2]

Test procedure: Finger and thumb opposition test

Test position: standing

- Stand with feet or heels together.
- Bend the elbow of one arm so that the forearm and hand are held out in front at a 90° angle with the palm of the hand facing the child. The opposite arm should hang loosely by the side (Figure 2.5a).
- Bend the thumb and first finger to form a circle with the tip of the thumb and forefinger (Figure 2.5b).
- Open and close the circle between the thumb and forefinger using the tip of the thumb and finger five times.
- Repeat the movement five times using the tip of the thumb and the tip of the second (middle) finger. Continue the sequence with the remaining two fingers.
- Return the arm to a resting position alongside the body.
- Repeat the test sequence using the other hand.

Observations

1. Do the fingers of the opposite hand also move, that is, do they 'mirror' the movements of the active hand? If so, how much and with which fingers?
2. Is the child able to make the sequential movements with each finger?

(a)

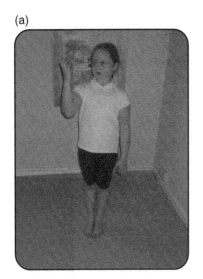

Figure 2.5a Dysdiadochokinesia fingers start position.

(b)

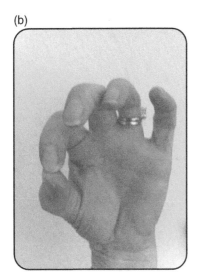

Figure 2.5b Thumb and finger opposition.

3. Does the child have difficulty with clarity of movements in one or several fingers? Which ones?
4. Does the child lose the ability to make the tip of the finger 'hit' the tip of the thumb?
5. Are the finger movements accompanied by movements of the mouth?

Scoring

Score separately for each hand:

0. No abnormality detected.
1. Slight mirroring of the fingers of the opposite hand.
2. More noticeable mirroring of the fingers of the opposite hand and clarity of movement in one finger may be poor.
3. Definite mirroring of the fingers of the opposite hand. The ability to juxtapose the fingertip and the tip of the thumb is lost. Impairment in articulation of independent movements in several fingers.
4. The child was unable to carry out the task.

2.4 Tests for Primitive Reflexes

Asymmetrical Tonic Neck Reflex (ATNR)

There are a variety of tests available to test for the continued presence of the ATNR. In young babies, the reflex is assessed in the supine position (lying on the back) with the tester gently rotating the head to each side. Head rotation elicits extension of the limbs on the jaw side and flexion of the occipital limbs up to six months of age.

The supine test is suitable for use with very young children or individuals with physical handicap. However, as muscle tone develops, the ATNR can be 'masked' by alteration in the general level of muscle tension held during testing, and for this reason, the supine test is not included in the screening test for this age group. More sensitive tests for eliciting the ATNR in older children (above six years of age) and adults include the quadruped test (Ayres[25]) and the Hoff–Schilder test.[26]

In the quadruped test, the child is instructed to go on hands and knees in a 'table' position (Figure 2.6a and Figure 2.6b) with the back of the head held level with the spine. The tester gently rotates the head as far as possible to one side. If the ATNR is present as the head is turned, flexion will occur in the *occipital* arm. The reflex may be present on one side only or differ in strength on either side. The tester observes the degree of flexion in the occipital arm when the head is turned to either side.

The ATNR is scored in the direction to which the head is turned. That is, when the head is turned to the right, the tester will observe the degree of flexion in the *left* occipital arm; if flexion in the occipital side is observed, the tester will record the degree of flexion as evidence of the ATNR being present to the *right*.

It should be noted that some studies have found that the ATNR can be elicited in normal primary (elementary) school children up to the age of eight years on the quadruped test, with younger children (six years of age) showing more evidence of the reflex than children at eight years of age. One study concluded that flexion of the elbow up to 30° on the occipital side could be considered normal in children up to eight years of age,[27] while Silver found the presence of the ATNR to be stronger in children over five years of age with maturational lag and emotional and reading disorders.[28] Others have found the ATNR to be stronger in children aged from seven to nine years with dyslexia compared to able readers.[29] Bearing this in mind, results of the quadruped test should be used *qualitatively* in children under eight years of age with medium to high scores only providing an indication of neuromotor immaturity likely to interfere with the physical aspects of handwriting, hand–eye coordination and tasks that involve crossing the midline.

The Hoff–Schilder test, carried out in the erect position (sometimes referred to as the arm extension test), is suitable for children from seven years of age but should be interpreted cautiously when used with children under seven years of age. Under eight years of age, the younger the child, the more easily the ATNR can be elicited because the postural mechanisms of the child are less mature.

Test procedure: Ayres quadruped test for the ATNR[25]

Test position: hands and knees

Instruct the child to go on hands and knees into the 'table' or four-point kneeling position (Figure 2.6a):

(a)

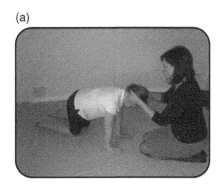

Figure 2.6a ATNR Ayres start position.

(b)

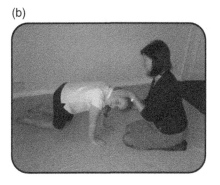

Figure 2.6b ATNR Ayres head rotation.

- The tester kneels in front of the subject and slowly rotates his/her head to one side, keeping the head parallel to the shoulder line (Figure 2.6b); when rotated, pause in this position for 5–10 seconds.
- Return the head to the midline; pause for 5–10 seconds.
- Turn the head to the opposite side; pause for 5–10 seconds.
- Return to the midline; pause for 5–10 seconds.
- Repeat the sequence four times. If the result is markedly positive on the first or second rotation, it is not necessary to repeat the procedure four times.

Observations

As the subject's head is turned to one side, is there flexion in the opposite arm, shoulder or hip?

Score the reflex as positive on the side to which the head is turned if present.

Scoring

0. No movement of the opposite arm, shoulder or hip (**no reflex present**).
1. Slight bending of the opposite arm or movement of the shoulder or hip (**reflex present up to 25%**).
2. Definite bending of the opposite arm or movement of the shoulder or hip (**reflex present up to 50%**).
3. Marked bending of the opposite arm, with or without shoulder or hip involvement (**reflex present up to 75%**).
4. Collapse of the occipital arm as a result of head rotation. There may also be hip involvement (**reflex 100% retained in the arm on the side to which the head is turned**).

Adapted Hoff–Schilder test for the ATNR (from seven years of age[30])

Test procedure

Test position

(c)

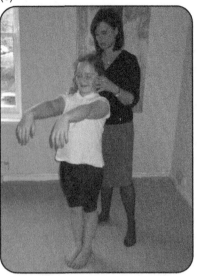

Figure 2.6c ATNR Schilder test start position for adapted Hoff–Schilder test.

(d)

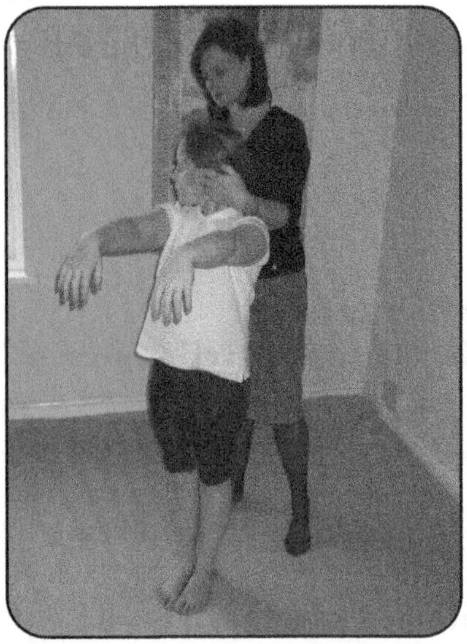

Figure 2.6d ATNR Schilder head rotation.

Erect, feet together and arms extended at shoulder height to the front with wrists flexed and eyes closed. Tester stands behind the test subject (Figure 2.6c).

The subject is instructed to 'Stand with your feet together, arms stretched out at shoulder height and wrists floppy.* Close your eyes. I am going to turn your head to each side, but I want your arms to remain where they are.'

The tester should demonstrate the required position of the arms during rotation of the head before applying the test:

- Slowly rotate the head to one side (Figure 2.6d).
- Pause for 5–10 seconds.
- Slowly return the head to the midline.
- Pause for 5–10 seconds.
- Slowly rotate the head to the other side.
- Repeat the sequence from two to three times.
- Repeat once more, turning the head quickly (but carefully).

If there is pain or resistance when rotating the head, do *not* continue to rotate the head beyond this point.

Observations

- Note any movement of the arm(s) *in the direction of head rotation* or counter-movement of the hips. The latter might indicate retention of the ATNR in the legs.
- Note any gravitational insecurity as a result of closing the eyes on head rotation.
- Is balance affected? This can be as a result of vestibular stimulation and/or residual presence of the ATNR in the legs.

*The original Hoff–Schilder test does not include the instructions to have wrists flexed and hands relaxed. INPP included this adaptation as some test subjects extend the hands during the test making it easier to maintain control of the arm position when the head is rotated and obscuring the true extent of the reflex.

Scoring

Score the reflex on the side to which the head is being turned:

0. No movement of the arms in response to head rotation
1. Slight deviation of the arm(s) up to 12–15° in the direction of head rotation
2. 30° rotation of the arms
3. 45° rotation of the arms
4. 90° rotation of the arms

The Symmetrical Tonic Neck Reflex (STNR)

In the infant, flexion of the head in the quadruped position will elicit bending of the arms and extension of the legs; extension of the head in the quadruped position will elicit extension of the arms and flexion in the legs.

To test for the presence of the STNR, the child is instructed to go on hands and knees in the 'table' position and to look upwards 'as if looking towards the ceiling', arching the head (not the back) upwards and backwards. If the reflex is present in extension as the head is lifted, the legs bend either pulling the buttocks towards the heels or the heels towards the buttocks, and the arms straighten (Figure 1.4 and Figure 1.5).

The child is then instructed to look down 'as if looking between your knees'. If the reflex is present in flexion as the head is flexed, the arms will bend (Figure 1.6) and there may also be elevation of the feet.

Test procedure: Symmetrical Tonic Neck Reflex

Test position: hands and knees

Instruct the child to go on hands and knees in the four-point kneeling 'table' position (Figure 2.7a):

- The child is instructed to maintain the test position in the arms and the legs and to slowly bend the head down *as if looking between your knees keeping your arms straight and the rest of the body still* (Figure 2.7b).
- Hold the position for five seconds and then slowly move the head upwards *as if looking at the ceiling* (Figure 2.7c). Repeat up to six times.

Observations

- Note any bending of the arms or raising of the feet as a result of head flexion.
- Flexion in the lower body as a result of head extension.
- Note any attempt to alter the hand position or 'locking' of the elbows during testing or arching and hollowing of the back. Arching and hollowing of the back may be an attempt to deflect the effect of the reflex but is not necessarily a sign of the STNR being present.
- Scoring for signs of the STNR in flexion and extension are listed as follows:

(a)

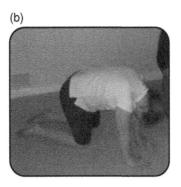

Figure 2.7a STNR start position.

(b)

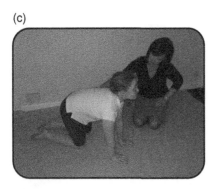

Figure 2.7b STNR test with head flexion.

(c)

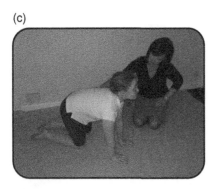

Figure 2.7c STNR test with head extension.

Scoring

(a) Flexion

    0. No response
    1. Tremor in one or both arms in response to flexion of the head
    2. Slight bending of the elbows
    3. Definite bending of the arms as a result of head flexion and/or elevation of the feet
    4. Arms collapse when the head is flexed

(b) Extension

    0. No response
    1. Slight movement in the hips (flexion in the lower body)
    2. Small movement in the hips
    3. Definite movement in the hips
    4. Movement of the bottom back onto the ankles so that the child is in the 'sitting cat' position

Tonic Labyrinthine Reflex (TLR): Erect test

In the infant, movement of the head through the mid-plane (flexion or extension of the head) will elicit changes in body position and muscle tonus.

When tested in infants and very young children, the test is usually carried out in the suspended supine position. However, as with the ATNR, as children develop postural control and muscle tone, the reflex can be inhibited in positions where there is minimal challenge to balance and posture, for example, when lying down, but fails to be inhibited as the tension and tone required to maintain posture and balance increase. An additional test for the TLR has been developed for use beyond the infancy period to assess the presence of the TLR in the erect (upright) position.

The child is instructed to stand with feet together and arms by the sides with the eyes closed and to slowly tilt the head back 'as if looking towards the ceiling'. If the reflex is present in extension, either movement of the head as it passes through the mid-plane or when the head is in an extended position, will result in significant increase in extensor muscle tonus throughout the body.

The child is then instructed to slowly bring the head forwards 'as if looking down at your toes'. If the reflex is present in flexion as the head is moved forwards through the mid-plane into flexion, there will be significant increase in flexor muscle tonus affecting the entire length of the body.

As distribution of muscle tone is involved in the control of both balance and posture, if the reflex is present in either position, head movement through the mid-plane can interfere with control of upright balance as a result of the influence on muscle tone.

(a)

Traces of the tonic labyrinthine reflex can persist under different postural conditions up to 3½ years of age but should be suppressed from this time.

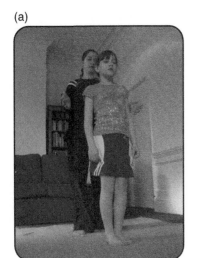

Figure 2.8a TLR test position.

Test procedure: Tonic Labyrinthine Reflex

Test position: standing

Please note it is important for the tester to stand behind or beside the child throughout the test procedure, as movement of the head can result in loss of balance.

Instruct the subject to stand with feet together and arms straight at the sides of the body. Tester stands behind the subject (Figure 2.8a):

- Slowly tilt the head back into an extended position, *as if looking up at the ceiling*, and then instruct the subject to close the eyes (Figure 2.8b). (Stand behind to support in case of loss of balance.)

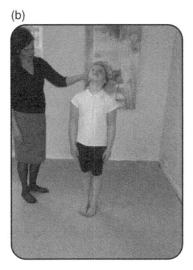

Figure 2.8b TLR erect test head extension.

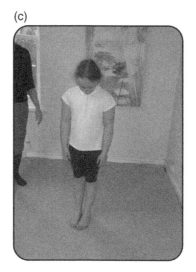

Figure 2.8c TLR erect test head flexion.

- Slowly move the head forwards, *as if looking down at the toes*, and maintain that position for a further 10 seconds (Figure 2.8c).
- Repeat the sequence from three to four times.

Observations

- Note any loss of balance or alteration of balance which results from flexion or extension of the head through the mid-plane.
- Observe any compensatory changes in muscle tone at the back of the knees or gripping or increased extensor tone in the toes which occurs when the head is moved through the mid-plane.
- Ask the child how he/she feels immediately after testing, and note any comments about feelings of dizziness or nausea during the testing – both of which might indicate faulty vestibular–proprioceptive interaction and/or the residual presence of the tonic labyrinthine reflex.

Scoring

0. No response.
1. Slight alteration of balance and muscle tone as a result of change in head position.
2. Impairment of control of balance during test and/or alteration of muscle tone.
3. Near loss of balance and/or alteration of muscle tone and/or disorientation as a result of test procedure.
4. Loss of balance and/or marked adjustment in muscle tone in attempt to stabilize balance. This may be accompanied by dizziness or nausea.

The Moro reflex

The Moro reflex is assessed shortly after birth and during routine developmental checks in the first four months. The test used with infants involves placing the infant in the supine position with head supported and then either lowering the head or slapping the supporting surface.

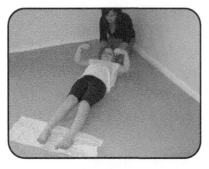

Figure 2.9 Moro reflex standard test start position.

Older children, who have developed muscle tone, may try to control the reflex reaction in this position by increasing extensor tone. For this reason, the test has been adapted for use with older children, requiring them to hold the arms in the air with the wrists flexed (Figure 2.9) and to maintain this position when the head is lowered. If the reflex is present, involuntary abduction can be observed in the arms when the head is lowered.

Standard test (adapted by Goddard Blythe for use with children and adults, 2003)[31]

Test procedure

Test position

- Supine with a small cushion placed under the middle of the back at shoulder level
- Legs slightly bent at the knees resting on the heels with feet apart
- Arms flexed and held up as if getting ready to clasp a large ball but with wrists flexed
- Head supported by the tester, slightly flexed and supported above the level of the spine
- Eyes closed as in Figure 2.9

Instruction

In a few moments time, I am going to let your head drop back a little way. I promise your head will not hit the floor. I want you to try to keep the rest of your body still in the test position.

- When the subject's head is relaxed, supported by the tester's hands, the tester drops the head at least 2 in. (5 cm) below the level of the spine, always keeping the hands beneath the subject's head so that the head is caught **before** it touches the floor.

Observations

- Can the subject maintain the arm position when the head drops or is there abduction of the arms?
- How much abduction of the arms do you observe?
- Is the subject visibly distressed by the procedure (over-arousal)?
- Is there a marked alteration in subject's colour following the procedure, that is, pallor or reddening of the skin?
- Is the subject very quiet or withdrawn following the test procedure?
- Is the subject unable to relax the neck muscles to allow the head to drop?

Scoring

0. No movement of the arms and no sign of distress or discomfort
1. Fractional movement of the arms outwards (abduction) or momentary freeze
2. Definite arm involvement and slight freeze reaction and/or signs of emotional discomfort following test procedure
3. Partial abduction of the arms and dislike of test procedure
4. Abduction of the arms and/or visibly distressed by the test procedure

If the subject is unable to 'let go' for the head to drop, this *might* suggest the Moro reflex is present.

2.5 Sample Score Sheets

Child assessment

Date	1st assessment	2nd assessment
Name Code number Age of subject		
1. Neuromotor tests		
Romberg test (eyes open)	0 1 2 3 4	0 1 2 3 4
Romberg test (eyes closed)	0 1 2 3 4	0 1 2 3 4
One-leg stand (right leg)	0 1 2 3 4	0 1 2 3 4
One-leg stand (left leg)	0 1 2 3 4	0 1 2 3 4
Thumb and finger opposition (right hand)	0 1 2 3 4	0 1 2 3 4
Thumb and finger opposition (left hand)	0 1 2 3 4	0 1 2 3 4
Asymmetrical tonic neck reflex (right) – quadruped test	0 1 2 3 4	0 1 2 3 4
Asymmetrical tonic neck reflex (left) – quadruped test	0 1 2 3 4	0 1 2 3 4
Asymmetrical tonic neck reflex (right) – adapted Hoff–Schilder test	0 1 2 3 4	0 1 2 3 4
Asymmetrical tonic neck reflex (left) – adapted Hoff–Schilder test	0 1 2 3 4	0 1 2 3 4
Symmetrical tonic neck reflex (flexion)	0 1 2 3 4	0 1 2 3 4
Symmetrical tonic neck reflex (extension)	0 1 2 3 4	0 1 2 3 4
Tonic labyrinthine reflex (flexion)	0 1 2 3 4	0 1 2 3 4
Tonic labyrinthine reflex (extension)	0 1 2 3 4	0 1 2 3 4
Moro reflex standard test	0 1 2 3 4	0 1 2 3 4
Total – neuromotor tests	**/60**	**/60**
Percentage score: total/60 × 100		

2.6 Sample Observation Sheets

(Additional score and observation sheets can be downloaded from http://www.inpp.org.uk/scoresheets)

Child assessment

Date	1st assessment	2nd assessment
Name Code number Age of child		
1. *Neuromotor tests*		
Romberg test (eyes open)		
Romberg test (eyes closed)		
One-leg stand (right leg)		
One-leg stand (left leg)		
Thumb and finger opposition (right hand)		
Thumb and finger opposition (left hand)		
Asymmetrical tonic neck reflex (right) – quadruped test		
Asymmetrical tonic neck reflex (left) – quadruped test		
Asymmetrical tonic neck reflex (right) – adapted Hoff–Schilder test		
Asymmetrical tonic neck reflex (left) – adapted Hoff–Schilder test		
Symmetrical tonic neck reflex (flexion)		
Symmetrical tonic neck reflex (extension)		
Tonic labyrinthine reflex (flexion)		
Tonic labyrinthine reflex (extension)		
Moro reflex standard test		

2.7 Interpreting the Scores

Children

The final scores have been divided into different sections to identify whether signs of immaturity are more prevalent in one or several areas of functioning.

Scores are interpreted in five categories:

1. No Abnormality Detected (NAD)
2. **Low** score < 25%
3. **Medium** score 25–49%
4. **High score** 50–74%
5. **Very high score** 75–100%

Tests for gross muscle coordination and balance

1	NAD	No action required
2	Low score	INPP school programme indicated
3	Medium score	Further assessment by an INPP practitioner and INPP individual programme indicated
4	High score	INPP assessment and INPP individual programme indicated
5	Very high score	Referral for further medical investigations indicated. Following appropriate assessment, an INPP programme may also be of benefit *Please note that although an individual programme is recommended if scores fall in the medium to high range, children will also benefit from participating in the INPP school programme if for family or financial reasons they are unable to access an individual assessment and an individual remedial programme*

Tests for aberrant reflexes

1	NAD	No action required
2	Low score	INPP school programme indicated
3	Medium score	Further assessment by an INPP practitioner and INPP individual programme indicated. (INPP school programme will be of benefit if access to an individual programme is not available)
4	High score	INPP assessment and INPP individual programme indicated
5	Very high score	Referral for further medical investigations indicated. Following appropriate assessment and recommendations, an INPP programme may also be of benefit *Please note that although an individual programme is recommended if scores fall in the medium to high range, children will also benefit from participating in the INPP school programme if for family or financial reasons they are unable to access an individual assessment and an individual remedial programme*

If a test subject is unable to complete the Romberg test together with a fully retained ATNR, an additional test for the Babinski reflex should be carried out. If all three signs are abnormal, the patient should be referred for further neurological investigations.

References

1   De Quirós, JB and Schrager, O (1979) *Neuropsychological fundamentals in learning disabilities.* Academic Therapy Publications, Novato, CA.

2   Kohen Raz, R (1986) *Learning disabilities and postural control.* Freund Publishing House, London.

3   Sparto, PJ, Redfern, MS, Jasko, JG, Casselbrant, ML, Mandel, EM and Furman, JM (2006) The influence of dynamic visual cues for postural control in children aged 7-12 years. *Experimental Brain Research,* **168**(4): 505–516.

4   Barela, JA, Jeka, JJ and Clark, JE (2003) Postural control in children: coupling to dynamic somatosensory information. *Experimental Brain Research,* **150**(4): 434–442.

5   Forssberg, H and Nashner, LM (1982) Ontogenetic development of postural control in man: adaptation to altered support and visual conditions during stance. *Journal of Neuroscience,* **2**(5): 545–552.

6   Shumway-Cook, A and Woollacott, M (1985) The growth of stability: postural control from a developmental perspective. *Journal of Motor Behavior,* **17**(2): 131–147.

7   Taguchi, K and Tada, C (1988) Change of body sway with group of children. In: Amblard, B, et al. (eds), *Posture and gait: development adaptation and modulation.* Elsevier, Amsterdam. pp. 59–65.

8   Shumway-Cook, A and Woollacott, M (2001) *Motor control: theory and practical applications.* Lippincott Williams & Wilkins, Baltimore, MD.

9   Foudriat, BA, Di Fabio, P and Anderson, JH (1993) Sensory organization of balance responses in children 3–6 years of age: a normative study with diagnostic implications. *International Journal of Pediatric Otorhinolaryngology,* **27**(3): 255–271.

10 Morioka, S (2001) Changes in the ability to stand on one leg from babyhood to school age. *Rigakuryhogaku,* **28**: 325–328.

11 Morioka, S, Fukumoto, T, Hiyamizu, M, Matsuo, A, Takebayashi, H and Miyamoto, K (2012) Changes in the equilibrium of standing on one leg at various life stages. *Current Gerontology and Geriatrics Research,* **2012**: 1–6.

12 Schrager, OL (2000) Postural adaptive reactions in one-leg position depending upon normal and abnormal vestibular-proprioceptive-oculomotor-visual integration. Bases for clinical assessment of learning disabled children. Paper presented at the 14th European Conference of Neuro-Developmental Delay in Children with Specific Learning Difficulties, Chester. March 2000.

13 Schrager, O (1994/1999) Tonic postural reactions and language development. Towards a neuropsychological model of dysphasic disorders. Doctoral dissertation. PhD program in *"Cognition and its Disorders".* Department of Basic Psychology. School of Psychology. Autonomous University of Madrid/UAM, Madrid, Spain.

14 Drillien, CM and Drummond, MB (1977) *Neurodevelopmental problems in early childhood.* Blackwell Scientific Publications, Oxford.

15 Griffiths, TD, Sigmundsson, T, Takei, N, Rowe, D and Murray, RM (1998) Neurological abnormalities in familial and sporadic schizophrenia. *Brain,* **121**: 191–203.

16 Heinrichs, DW and Buchanan, RW (1988) Significance and meaning of neurological signs in schizophrenia. *American Journal of Psychiatry,* **145**: 11–18.

17 Fellick, JM, Thomson, APJ, Sills, J and Hart, CA (2001) Neurological soft signs in mainstream pupils. *Archives of Disease in Childhood,* **85**: 371–374.

18 Mutti, M, Sterling, HM and Spalding, NV (1978) *QNST Quick Neurological Screening Test,* Revised edn. Academic Therapy Publications, Novato, CA.

19 Fog, E and Fog, M (1963) Cerebral inhibition examined by associated movements. In: Mac Keith, R and Bax, M (eds), *Minimal cerebral dysfunction*. Papers from the International Study Group held at Oxford, September 1962. William Heinemann Medical Books Ltd., London.

20 Accardo, PJ (1980) *A neuro-developmental perspective on specific learning difficulties*. University Park Press, Baltimore, MD.

21 Kuhlman, F (1939) *Tests of mental development*. Educational Test Bureau, Minneapolis, MN.

22 Touwen, BCL (1970) *Examination of the child with minor neurological dysfunction*. William Heinemann Medical Books, London.

23 Grant, WW, Boelshce, AN and Zin, D (1973) Developmental patterns of two motor functions. *Developmental Medicine & Child Neurology*, **15**: 171–177.

24 Satz, P, Taylor, HG, Friel, J and Fletcher, JM (1978) Some developmental and predictive precursors of reading disabilities. A six year follow-up. In: Benton, AL and Pearl, D (eds), *Dyslexia: an appraisal of current knowledge*. Oxford University Press, New York.

25 Ayres, AJ (1978) *Sensory integration and learning disorders*. Western Psychological Services, Los Angeles, CA.

26 Hoff, H and Schilder, P (1927) *Die Lagereflexe des Menschen. Klinische Untersuchungen über Haltungs- und Stellreflexe und verwandte Phänomene*. Julius Springer, Wien.

27 Parmentier, CL (1975) The asymmetrical tonic neck reflex in normal first and third grade children. *The American Journal of Occupational Therapy*, **29**(8): 463–468.

28 Silver, AA (1952) Postural and righting responses in children. *Journal of Pediatrics*, **41**: 493–498.

29 McPhillips, M and Jordan Black, JA (2007) Primary reflex persistence in children with reading difficulties (dyslexia): a cross-sectional study, *Neuropsychologia*, **45**: 748–754.

30 Critchley, M (1970) *The dyslexic child*. Heinemann Medical Books, London.

31 Goddard Blythe, SA (2003) Adaptation to the standard test for assessing presence of the Moro reflex in school aged children and adults. INPP Supervision Days. December 2003. Chester

3
Neuromotor Immaturity in Adults

Problems associated with neuromotor immaturity are not confined to the childhood years. As children mature, the nervous system continues to change and develop, but if problems linked to immature reflexes, vestibular functioning and postural reactions remain, associated problems tend to grow up with them, as traits or 'threads', which become woven into the fabric of the personality.

One of the reasons for this is that if lower brain centres normally employed in the sub-conscious aspects of the basic functions of posture, balance, control of movement and perception do not function efficiently, higher cortical centres must be recruited to compensate. This can result in cortical 'overload' with effect upon cognitive processing, cognitive attribution and somatic affect. It can also increase arousal levels to normally non-noxious stimuli so that the autonomic nervous system reacts *before* frontal areas of the brain process the information resulting in somatic reactions preceding and temporarily overwhelming cortical control. 'If there is a conflict between feelings and logic and feelings are too strong, feelings will tend to win'.[1]

3.1 The Role of the Vestibular System and Its Connections

The vestibular system, or balance system, is the main gravity sensor.

It provides the dominant input about an individual's movement and orientation in space. Together with the cochlea, the auditory organ, it is situated in the vestibulum in the inner ear. The receptor organ consists of two fluid-filled sacs, the *utricle* and *saccule* (otoliths), and three semi-circular canals, which lie perpendicular to each other and represent the three spatial planes. Suspended in the fluid (endolymph) are specialized receptor cells – hair cells – which are sensitive to fluid currents. When there is a shift or change of position of the head, the *endolymph* is set in motion which stimulates the receptors, transmitting the information to the brain, which then sets off appropriate reflex responses.

The two otolithic organs on each side comprise the utricle and the saccule. Otoconia crystals in the *otoconia layer* rest on a viscous gel layer and are heavier than their surroundings. During

Neuromotor Immaturity in Children and Adults: The INPP Screening Test for Clinicians and Health Practitioners, First Edition. Sally Goddard Blythe.
© 2014 John Wiley & Sons, Ltd. Published 2014 by John Wiley & Sons, Ltd.

linear acceleration, they are displaced which in turn deflects the hair cells, thereby producing a sensory signal. Most of the utricular signals elicit eye movements, while the majority of the saccular signals project to muscles that control our posture.

Signals from the inner ear pass to the brain and enter the brainstem, where they terminate in four vestibular nuclei that serve different functions in communicating vestibular information to other parts of the central nervous system via five major connections:

1. Vestibular–spinal system, which innervates reflexes that act on the trunk and limbs to maintain equilibrium.
2. Vestibular–Ocular Reflex (VOR), which is responsible for stabilizing an observed object on the retina while moving the head. When the head moves, the VOR responds with an eye movement that is equal in magnitude but opposite in direction, thereby stabilizing the visual image on the retina. Head movement triggers an inhibitory signal to the extra-ocular muscles on one side and an excitatory signal to the muscles on the other side, resulting in a compensatory movement of the eyes. (Position of the head in relation to the body and to the supporting surface is important for the optimal functioning of this reflex.)
3. Vestibular–cerebellar connections, which compare input from the visual, vestibular and proprioceptive systems and mediate changes in the VOR.

(While the vestibular nuclear complex is the primary processor of vestibular input and implements direct, fast connections between incoming afferent information and motor output neurons, the cerebellum is the adaptive processor; it monitors vestibular performance and readjusts central vestibular processing if necessary. At both locations, vestibular sensory input is processed in association with somatosensory and visual sensory input.[2])

4. Vestibular cortex, which contributes to *perception* of position in space, body schema and self-coherence.[3]
5. Accessory pathway – based on information received from the otoliths concerning absolute position of the head in space. This operates via the XIth *accessory cranial nerve* to innervate the trapezius and sternomastoid neck muscles to keep the head upright despite changes in body position.

Each of these pathways forms a continuous feedback loop which contributes to the collective functioning of pathways involved in providing vital information to other parts of the brain concerning body position and to facilitate stability and equilibrium. Together, they provide the physical basis for stable perception represented as a functional model in Figure 3.1.

Other vestibular reflexes and systems involved include the vestibulocollic reflex and reticulospinal system. The vestibulocollic reflex is indicative of otolithic (saccular) function and can be elicited by direct stimulation of the inferior vestibular nerve, acoustic stimuli, mechanical stimulation of the forehead and galvanic stimulation.[4] Action of the vestibulocollic reflex stabilizes the head in relation to the body, while the vestibular spinal reflexes act on the trunk and limbs[5]:

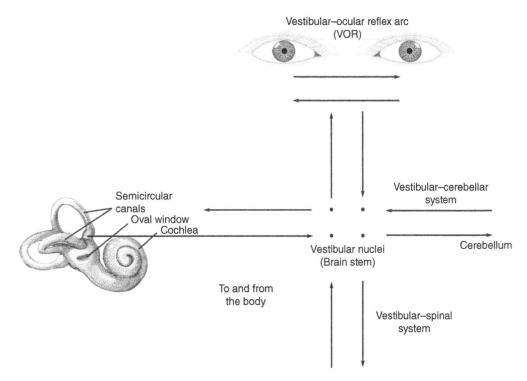

Figure 3.1 Functional links to and from the vestibular system. © Sally Goddard Blythe, 2005.

The *reticulospinal tract* receives sensory input from all of the vestibular nuclei as well as from all of the other sensory and motor systems involved with maintaining balance. This projection has both crossed and uncrossed components and is very highly collateralized. As a result, the reticulospinal tract through the entire extent of the spinal cord is poorly defined, but it is probably involved in most balance reflex motor actions, including postural adjustments made to extra-vestibular sensory input (auditory, visual and tactile stimuli).[2]

Connections to the Reticular Activating System (RAS) are relevant in the context of anxiety and panic disorder because the RAS is involved in arousal and many of the physical sensations associated with anxiety.

Blythe[6] first suggested a physiological link between vestibular dysfunction, the RAS and feelings of anxiety in 1990. Others have mooted a similar pathway to anxiety describing how feelings of anxiety arise when the brain's arousal system produces a level of excitation that is higher than that which would usually be caused by the stimuli an individual is experiencing:

> The purpose of the arousal system is to ensure that an organism will switch into an 'alert mode', in which the individual is motivated to determine the environmental origin of the heightened arousal level, and resolve the issue in order to lower arousal back to an optimum level for normal (non-emergency) functioning. However, if the heightened arousal level is considerable, and essentially a false alarm (due to a functional defect in arousal regulation), the individual is likely to experience a vague, unpleasant, unlocalizable feeling, commonly known as anxiety.[7]

Why the vestibular system is implicated in hyper-arousal and anxiety is explained in the context of its role in contributing to gravitational security and a firm reference point in space.

Berthoz described the human relationship with gravity as being the one whereby:

> Gravity provides an ingenious frame of reference for indicating a 'vertical' uniformly distributed over the surface of the earth. This 'plumb line' is used by the sensors for angular acceleration of the head (semicircular canals). In this way the brain constantly keeps track of the absolute angle of the head in space, a veritable 'inertial guidance system' similar to the ones onboard aeroplanes and missiles to stabilise their position in flight. In humans, locomotion is not organised from the feet up. My theory is that coordination of multiple degrees of freedom of the limbs during locomotion is organised from the head, which is stabilised in rotation and constitutes an inertial guidance platform. This top-down control acts as a mobile frame of reference and liberates terrestrial animals from the ground.

He goes on to say:

> The vestibular system is not only a frame of reference for stabilizing the head and coordinating movements of the limbs. It is also critical to our perception of space and for constructing our bodies vis-à-vis the world.[3]

In theory, disorganization in the functioning of this system is not confined to disorientation but may also contribute to feelings of unreality – of literally being 'spaced out' – and body dysmorphia.

3.2 Historical Background to Links Between Vestibular–Cerebellar Dysfunction and Anxiety, Agoraphobia and Panic Disorder

The theory that there might be a relationship between vestibular, cerebellar and postural dysfunctions and agoraphobia and anxiety states is not new. In 1804, Joseph Mason Cox published a book *Practical Observations in Insanity*,[8] in which he described the use of new techniques using twisting, swinging and rotation of patients in a specially designed chair for the treatment of patients at the Fishponds Lunatic Asylum, near Bristol, which he found initially induced symptoms of pallor, nausea, vomiting and enuresis, followed by quiescence and sleep.

In 1870, Benedikt,[9] and, a few years later, Lannois and Tournier[10] suggested that agoraphobia might be of vestibular origin. In 1916, Bauer observed that certain cases of neurosis were accompanied by abnormal vestibular-cerebellar signs[11]; Leidler and Loewy[12] found spontaneous nystagmus to be present in 64 out of 78 cases of patients diagnosed with neurosis together with turning perceptions in the head and visual illusions of objects turning, and in 1933, neurologist Paul H. Schilder linked abnormal vestibular functioning to vegetative symptoms of nausea, dizziness and abnormal perception of heat and cold, concluding that 'probably the psyche can act on the vestibular system in a double way either affecting the nervous regulation directly or affecting it via vasomotor innervation of the labyrinth.'[13]

Von Weizsäcker[14] observed that every organic disease brings with it a pattern of psychic reactions – or that every organ has a corresponding psychic representation – and that, in effect, organic disease neurotizes the individual. Goldstein[15] was of the opinion that there are motor tendencies throughout the body that can disrupt the unity of the body unless they are united under the influence of cerebellar function. He believed that postural and righting reactions are the *starting point* for postural and motor unity and that the vestibular apparatus acts as the head organ of kinaesthetic function, having representatives all over the body. This observation tallies with Schilder's conclusion that 'vestibular changes disrupt the unity of the postural model of the body.'[5]

Frank and Levinson[16,17] documented their observations of the relationship between Cerebellar–Vestibular (CV) dysfunction and fears/phobias as well as associated anxiety states. Levinson[18,19] found that CV-dysfunctioning dyslexic children and adults who were experimentally treated with CV-stabilizing anti-motion sickness and related medications unexpectedly reported significant improvements in their fears/phobias, anxiety and frustration levels, mood and self-esteem and occasionally even obsessive–compulsive symptoms (Frank and Levinson[16,17]; Levinson[18-20]).

The use of antihistamines in the prevention of motion sickness has been recognized since the post-war period when by chance a woman suffering from urticaria was treated with Dramamine, prescribed for its antihistamine effects. The patient, who had been a lifelong sufferer from car sickness, found that she was symptom-free while taking the drug.[21] Brand and Perry later found that the efficacy of the antihistamines was due not to their primary pharmacological antihistamine properties, but to their effect upon the central nervous system.[22]

By the 1960s, many investigators in the field of motion sickness had reached the conclusion that motion sickness is the product of particular types of sensory conflict, defined as:

> a condition of *sensory re-arrangement* in which motion information signalled by the vestibular receptors, the eyes, and non-vestibular proprioceptors, is at variance with the kinds of inputs that are expected on the basis of past experience (pp. 147–170).[21]

It was thought to result from a disturbance in the harmony or coherence, which normally exists between these receptors, and there may be two types of re-arrangement involved:

1. Inter-modality conflict – between the eyes and the vestibular receptors
2. Intra-modality or intra-labyrinthine conflict – between the semi-circular canals and the otoliths

This theory of motion sickness has now been extended to include conflict between any of the sensors involved in the perception of position and motion including proprioception and the mechanoreceptors involved in surface stability.

Abnormal tonic neck and labyrinthine reflexes can provide either signposts of conflict in the functioning of these systems *or* may contribute to sensations of motion sickness as a result of inefficient head righting reactions in response to passive motion (car, train, boat, etc.) or abnormal changes to muscle tone and postural control as a result of active rotation, flexion or extension of the head. Such reactions were described some years later as vestibular–proprioceptive, vestibular–visual or vestibular–proprioceptive–visual 'mismatch'.[23] In addition to providing indications of immaturity or disturbance in the functioning of vestibular–proprioceptive pathways, abnormal labyrinthine, tonic neck reflexes and righting reactions can affect visual perception and influence vaso-motor and other somatic functions. Retention of these reflexes may be either symptomatic *of* or contribute *to* symptoms of vestibular–cerebellar dysfunction.

In 1979, Blythe and McGlown[24] outlined the findings of nine years of research showing that the overall majority of children and adults seen by them who were suffering from psychoneurotic symptoms and syndromes, and particularly those patients who appeared to be resistant to the therapy of choice (recidivists), had a cluster of hitherto undetected CNS dysfunctions confirmed by tests which revealed retention of primitive reflexes and vestibular dysfunction. In adults, a history of CNS dysfunction could predispose them to develop symptoms of 'secondary' neuroses, particularly panic disorder and agoraphobia.

They also noted that many of the adults had for many years been able to compensate for these previously undetected and unrecognized dysfunctions, but because the law of compensation exacts a price, the price in these cases was exacted at the emotional level in emotional functioning:

> Children, adolescents and adults with neuromotor immaturity, together with those individuals who are currently compensating adequately for their undetected and unrecognised dysfunctions, are subsequently submitted to a higher internal stress – excitation level, together with concomitant lower stress tolerance threshold, which renders them more vulnerable to life stressors.[25] In this respect Le Winn[26] wrote that the effect of neurological impairment upon the individual is to place them in a chronic state of internal excitation whereby they will be reactive to normally non-noxious stimuli.[24]

In 1982, Blythe and McGlown published the result of a pilot study which had investigated the presence of neurological dysfunction in a sample of 23 adults diagnosed with agoraphobia. Tests had been carried out in three categories:

1. Gross muscle coordination and balance
2. Presence of aberrant primitive reflexes and postural reactions
3. Tests for oculo-motor and visual-perceptual problems

Over 95% of the sample had problems with static balance on the Romberg test and showed signs of increased physiological nystagmus on tests for oculo-motor functioning. More than 90% had evidence of the asymmetrical tonic neck reflex, over 75% had a residual tonic labyrinthine reflex and over 70% still had traces of the symmetrical tonic neck reflex.[27]

Levinson[28] investigated the relationship between chronic dizziness and vestibular function in 15 patients with panic disorder compared to 15 patients with chronic dizziness without panic disorder. Using neurotological screening for spontaneous positional nystagmus with head-shaking and head-thrust tests, an audiometric examination and electronystagmography with bithermal stimulation according to Freyss, tests revealed that a significantly higher number of patients with panic disorder and chronic dizziness showed pathological neurotological findings in comparison to subjects with chronic dizziness only (nine and two patients, respectively; $p < 0.05$). Levinson formulated the hypothesis that 'the complaint of dizziness in patients with panic disorder may be linked to a malfunction of the vestibular system and vestibular disorders may play a role in the pathophysiology of panic disorder' (Reproduced with permission of Ammons Scientific Ltd.).[28] He went on to describe some of the symptoms and possible underlying mechanisms, which he believed underlay his findings, as follows:

1. *Imbalance mechanisms*, which often led to fears of heights, bridges, steps, falling, tripping, escalators, walking across wide-open spaces or intersections as well as fears of dizziness and losing control.
2. *Dyscoordination mechanisms*, which triggered fears of driving, sports, swimming, water, running, writing, and speaking (especially in public or social circumstances) as well as fears of walking or navigating across a busy intersection with no one or nothing to hold on to while having to turn one's head and judge distance, speed, and direction of criss-crossing cars.
3. *Disturbances of muscle tone* such as 'jelly legs' often triggered or reinforced anxieties of walking alone for fear of falling and losing control. Even the head bobbing sometimes reported among those anxiety-disordered appeared to result from unstable tone within the head and neck support muscles.
4. *Impaired motion-processing* resulted in either 'motion-sickness' and/or motion-anxiety responses to specific motion vectors and so readily explained fears of moving elevators, escalators, trains, planes, buses, and even the motion characterizing walking, and/or the fears triggered by such movement-confining situations as standing, sitting or lying still, as well as confining and restricting crowds.
5. *Impaired proprioception* underlay and explained a series of body-image illusions which were often unconsciously displaced outward and experienced as the floor tipping, rocking etc.
6. *Disturbances in orientation (compass functions)* may result in disorientation, spatial-temporal confusion, and a corresponding fear of new places, new situations, getting lost, and traveling alone.
7. *Sensory overloading*, real or relative, may result in photophobic or acoustic 'crowd' phobias triggered by such visual signals as fluorescent light, sun, flickering, specific colours (occasionally relieved by tinted glasses), and such noise signals as screeching brakes, thunder, and 'loud' social gatherings. Specific tactile or steady (constant) emotional stimuli may result in contact and 'relationship or commitment phobias' and claustrophobic-like anxiety. Even olfactory, barometric, and related sensory stimuli were noted to be phobic triggers.
8. *Sensory deprivation*, real or relative, triggered by shielding environments such as rooms without windows, underwater, darkness, tunnels and subways, steel elevators, and crowds, may result in 'claustrophobic' anxiety.
9. *Perseveration mechanisms* may result in the repetitive thoughts and actions characterizing obsessions and compulsions as well as the inability to inhibit, erase, or forget traumatic experiences, including those triggered by anxiety or panic attacks.
10. *Disturbances in the regulation of anxiety* were analogous to (and often overlapping with) the mechanisms modulating 'typical' responses of motion sickness and tended to vary from exaggerated (panic) to absent (psychopathy), and repetitive or perseverative to singular episodes.
11. *Secondary destabilization* of the autonomic nervous system, dysautonomia (sweating, palpitations, temperature changes, etc.), and dysregulation of the reflex (swallowing

and breathing) centers in the medulla oblongata (Carr & Sheehan[29]) and the nucleus coeruleus (Redmond[30]; Redmond and Huang[31]) as well as the anticipatory anxiety triggered by cerebral cortical sensitization readily explained a host of secondary or associated anxiety-related symptoms.[12]

An independent study carried out by a clinical psychologist working at a hospital in Scotland investigated the incidence of abnormal reflexes in adults who had sought clinical treatment for anxiety disorder. Using tests selected from the INPP Test Battery, the researcher assessed 26 patients and 26 control subjects for the presence of aberrant reflexes. The results revealed a significant difference in the reflex test mean scores between the patients with anxiety and the control group, with the tonic labyrinthine reflex and under-developed head righting reflexes showing the highest abnormal scores in the anxiety group compared to the control group. The researcher commented that 'these reflexes are regarded as exerting an influence over sensory processing, to the extent that the individual's relationship with gravity cannot function adaptively. A variety of problems result, and include dysfunction of balance, coordination and proprioception, all governed by the central nervous system'.[32]

3.3 Vestibular Dysfunction: Cause or Effect?

One of the chief problems for the clinician is how to define whether presenting symptoms of anxiety, agoraphobia or panic disorder are secondary consequences of primary underlying vestibular or vestibular–cerebellar dysfunction or whether anxiety has resulted in increased sensitivity to vestibular sensations.

Yardley and Redfern[33] reviewed evidence for three mechanisms through which psychological factors might aggravate sensations of dizziness and interfere with recovery from balance disorders. One behavioural response to dizziness is to avoid activities and environments that provoke symptoms, preventing individuals from developing the skills and adaptations needed to cope with similar situations. This avoidance is a 'secondary' psychological response to a primary symptom. Conversely, anxiety and arousal can provoke hyperventilation, which results in increased heart rate, dizziness and feelings of derealization.[34] It has been shown that postural control deteriorates during hyperventilation[35] and that hyperventilation can induce nystagmus among patients with vestibular lesions.[36] Increased anxiety can also affect cognitive processes involved in orientation.[33]

3.4 Rationale for a Somatogenic/Psychosomatic Basis to Some Anxiety Disorders

In an overview of the literature investigating a relationship between balance disorders and phobic postural vertigo, Holmberg[37] summarized some of the conflicting findings:

> Yardley et al. failed to find definite vestibular abnormalities among patients with panic disorder with agoraphobia. However, results from posturography correlated with the patients' experiences of dizziness.[38] Jacob has described that patients with panic disorder with agoraphobia and

dizziness often have signs of vestibular dysfunction and impaired balance control.[39] Jacob has similarly described that patients with panic disorder with agoraphobia who also suffer from dizziness have difficulties stabilizing themselves confronted with poor visual and proprioceptive information (being on boats and on heights).[40,41] He argued that vestibular dysfunction leads to a reliance on non-vestibular channels for balance control, i.e., vision and proprioception. This leads to sensitivity in situations with conflicting stimuli. Patients with this sensitivity, named *space and motion discomfort*, have poorer postural control if proprioceptive information is reduced during posturography. Such a balance strategy is labelled surface dependence (pp. 48–65).[24]

Abnormal tonic neck, labyrinthine and head righting reactions disturb normal vestibular–proprioceptive functioning as a result of the movement of the head and neck or of the environment, which affect body position and call on normal righting reactions for stabilization. Vestibular–proprioceptive 'mismatch' can lead to over-reliance on visual processing for orientation or increased surface dependence. When either of these compensatory processes is compromised or if either system becomes overloaded by a plethora of conflicting environmental stimuli with inability to filter irrelevant stimuli, the ability to process information cognitively becomes temporarily impaired, arousal and anxiety levels increase, and in certain situations feelings of imminent catastrophe or panic are elicited.

The 'sense of "self" is grounded in our relationship with gravity. When balance is secure we are able not only to manoeuvre and navigate but also to have a basis for perceptual stability – the precursor of coherently processing the environment. Perceptual stability is dependent on synergy in the integration of sensory information'.[22]

Stability in space, described by A. Jean Ayres as gravitational security, is fundamental not only to postural stability but also to spatial, perceptual and emotional security. As described earlier, the sense of self, of 'I', begins with stability in space and involves coherence in multiple structural and functional relationships (Figure 3.2).

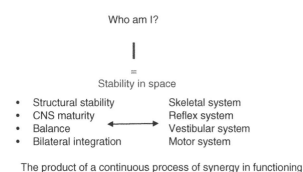

Figure 3.2 The sense of self – a continuous process of interaction between structure and function.

Balance is based on the integration in the CNS of sensory information in cooperation with continuously adapting motor responses towards the surrounding, which, in turn, supplies new sensory feedback. In addition to the vestibular system, it involves mechanoreceptors – pressure receptors in the skin – which provide information concerning the location of the body in relation to gravitational forces, particularly pressure receptors in the feet when standing, the sacral region when sitting and the hands and knees in the quadruped position; proprioceptors located in the muscles, tendons and joints, which provide information regarding the relationship between body position and body parts; and proprioceptors of the neck, which are important for location of the position of the head in relation to the trunk.

Retention of the Tonic Labyrinthine Reflex (TLR) can affect the functional relationship between the vestibular system, proprioceptive feedback derived from the neck and the body (vestibular–spinal system) and feedback derived from mechanoreceptors (supporting base), as a result of changes in muscle tone which occur in response to movement of the head through the mid-plane when standing.

Residual presence of the TLR is often linked to under-developed Head Righting Reflexes (HRRs), which can affect stability and control of eye movements involved in gaze control and underlying visual-perceptual disturbance. Empirical evidence based on patients seen at INPP over many years has indicated a consistent relationship between a retained TLR, under-developed HRRs and poor control of ocular convergence, resulting in a tendency to experience figure–ground effect. These clinical observations match patient description of fear induced by situations involving heights, escalators, crossing surfaces involving visual depth discrepancies (e.g. slatted bridge) and feelings of being overwhelmed in environments which involve processing multiple visual stimuli (supermarkets with banks of lights, stacked goods, etc. and city underground transport). While patients can usually name situations which provoke feelings of anxiety and panic, which they quickly learn to avoid, they do not recognize the *specific* environmental triggers to feelings of panic and tend to generalize fear or fear of fear to avoid *all* situations which might engender anxiety. This behavioural adaptation is consistent with Yardley et al.'s findings that patient avoidance hinders recovery[21] and Blythe's original theory that underlying physical dysfunction can lead to the development of 'secondary neuroses'.[15]

Similarly, retention of the Symmetrical Tonic Neck Reflex (STNR) normally elicited in the quadruped or sitting positions results in opposing reactions to changes in muscle tone in the upper and lower sections of the body in response to flexion or extension of the head, affecting truncal stability and posture.

In an unpublished study carried out by Bein-Wierzbinski[42] in which children were assessed for abnormal reflexes using standard neurological tests and for aberrant eye movements using a computerized infra-red eye tracking device, residual presence of the STNR was linked to immature *vertical* eye tracking movements. Vertical eye tracking is involved in the perception of heights, and problems with vertical eye tracking can interfere with the visual perception needed to function in environments that involve the perception of height, depth and motion (e.g. standing at the top of a moving escalator and stepping on and off).

The Asymmetrical Tonic Neck Reflex (ATNR) can result in feelings of instability in response to *lateral* rotation of the head. A common problem described by adults with agoraphobia seen at INPP is anxiety when a pedestrian is trying to cross a busy road. As this usually involves turning the head to either side several times to assess the presence and speed of oncoming traffic, head rotation can affect control of balance, elicit vestibular–proprioceptive mismatch and result in feelings of disorientation, difficulty judging timing and speed of fast-approaching objects and being able to coordinate a rapid response, eliciting feelings of anxiety and panic:

'While the vestibular organs provide the most important information regarding detection of head movement, activation of afferents from these receptors evoke the vestibulocollic reflex (VCR), which normally stabilises the head position in space'.[43] Retention of the ATNR can interfere with this process which, under normal conditions, 'acts on the neck musculature in order to stabilize the head. Reflex head movement counters the movement sensed by the otoliths or semicircular canals. The neural pathways mediating this reflex are as yet uncertain. Automatic body movements reflect overlay of several synergies – the main areas discussed in the classic literature are related to body positioning alone (basic postural reflexes and ones related to vestibular input – labyrinthine or vestibular spinal reflexes). When we stand or move, our body tends to automatically assume particular postures based on the *combination* of those responses' (pp. 147–170).[44]

The neck acts as a vital junction in synergetic functioning of these systems, normally unifying the relationship between head, body and visual perception. The efficiency of vestibulocollic reflexes has been shown to decline in adults with age.[45]

The presence of normal postural righting reactions, particularly Head Righting Reflexes (HRRs), is essential to this process. There are two types of HRR – Labyrinthine Head Righting Reflex (LHRR) and Oculo-head Righting Reflex (OHRR). HRRs develop gradually from birth over many months and must be re-calibrated in relation to the supporting surface each time a child learns a new postural skill (sitting, crawling, standing, walking, etc.).

3.5 Postural Righting Reactions

Labyrinthine Head Righting Reflexes (LHRRs)

The LHRR is elicited when an infant is supported and the body is tilted either forwards, backwards or to one side or by stimulation of the otoliths. As the LHRR develops, the infant will respond by bringing the head to the centre by adjusting the head position in equal proportion and in the opposite direction to the displacement of the body. The reflex comprises compensatory contraction of the neck muscles to keep the head level in the correct relationship with the body in relation to the supporting surface. As a result of this automatic adjustment of head position, the vestibular system operates from a stable reference point in relation to the supporting base for other postural adjustments to be made.

The labyrinthine head righting reflex responds to impulses that arise from the otolith of the labyrinth, combined with other centres in the *midbrain*, enabling the infant to maintain proper head alignment with the environment in the absence of other sensory (particularly visual) channels (e.g. in the dark).

The **oculo-head righting reflex** on the other hand responds to *visual* cues and is dependent on the functioning of the *cerebral cortex*. It maintains the head in a stable position and the eyes fixed on visual targets despite other movements of the body. This is necessary to focus the image on the fovea, for visual fixation and maintaining visual attention when the body is moving, and occurs as a result of neural connections between the eyes and the vestibular system (VOR). The VOR provides a mechanism whereby when the head moves in one direction, the eyes rotate in the direction opposite to the movement of the head. The timing of the opposing movement is essential for the target to remain fixated on the fovea, enabling vision to be sharp and clear. Jacobs[46] and Carpenter[47] showed that visual acuity declines by 50% at a point 2° from the centre of the fovea, enabling a person to visualize objects briefly during head movements.

Under-developed righting reactions affect adaptation of posture and balance to changing conditions which can affect gaze control. When a person with under-developed head righting reactions encounters an environment where multiple rapidly moving visual stimuli are present, he or she may have difficulty processing visual information, particularly filtering out irrelevant stimuli to maintain focus and orientation in space. During the period of disorientation, the cortex is temporarily unable to 'make sense' of multiple sensory stimuli; while cortical processing is temporarily disabled, lower brain centres including the limbic system alert the autonomic nervous system innervating biochemical changes in response to perceived threat (freeze, fight or flight). Such changes are experienced somatically and interpreted cognitively as fear.

Most people have experienced something of this phenomenon under either natural or contrived conditions. Consider, for example, what happens if you spin round very fast a number of times in one direction only. When body rotation stops, for a few seconds, the visual world appears to be moving and is blurred. This is because rapid rotation of the body has stimulated motion of fluid in the inner ear, which continues for a few moments after body rotation has stopped; the visual system cannot pinpoint the visual image on the fovea until the fluid has stabilized. During the period of 'dizziness' (meaning scatterbrained), physical symptoms such as nausea, increased heart rate, sweating and wobbly legs may be experienced. These are the same *physical* sensations that are felt under conditions of extreme anxiety. In this way, the physical sensations associated with anxiety can be produced by overstimulation or inappropriate stimulation of the vestibular system and associated pathways. Motion sickness also occurs as a result of a similar process, when movement in a particular plane or combination of planes disrupts the normal relationship between body, balance and vision.

The head righting reflexes are necessary to maintain congruence between body position, vestibular functioning and the eye movements involved in gaze control. If the head does not make the appropriate compensatory adjustment in response to displacement of the body or the environment, the vector from which eye movements take their cue is dislocated, affecting the position of the image on the fovea and also potentially affecting the angle and direction of eye movements.

3.6 The Moro Reflex: A Trigger for Panic?

(For a description of the Moro reflex in infancy and its possible effects on children and adults if retained, see 'The Moro Reflex' in Chapter 1).

In infancy (from birth to four months), the Moro reflex is primarily elicited as a result of stimulation of the labyrinth, particularly loss of head control (before more advanced postural reactions and muscle tone needed to support head control are present), but it is also sensitive to sudden unexpected sensory stimuli of any kind, including sudden change of position

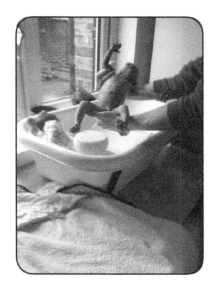

Figure 3.3 Moro reflex in reaction to sudden alteration of position and temperature in a neonate.

(Figure 3.3), loud noises, change of light, movement on the periphery of the visual field or rapid alteration of temperature. In normal development, the Moro reflex is inhibited at two to four months of age and coincides with development of early head righting reactions in prone and supine positions.

In adults presenting for assessment at INPP with anxiety and balance problems with evidence of the Asymmetrical Tonic Neck Reflex (ATNR), Tonic Labyrinthine Reflex (TLR) and under-developed head righting reactions, the Moro reflex can often be elicited using either the standard test (see 'Standard Test' in Chapter 4) or a test involving loss of balance (see 'Erect (Drag) Test for the Moro Reflex' in Chapter 4). This 'Moro' reaction, in contrast to a normal parachute reflex,* results in immediate symptoms of acute anxiety, disorientation and temporary emotional fragmentation, described by patients as being 'like having a panic attack'.

The Moro reflex is thought to form a part of a developmental chain of startle reflexes, which begin with a primitive 'freeze and withdrawal' reaction to aversive stimuli (like a rabbit startled by the headlights of an approaching car in the dark), followed by the Moro reflex (fight and flight) and eventually superseded by an adult 'startle' response (Strauss reflex).

The Strauss reflex is a startle response elicited by a sudden or unexpected stimulus. The original films of Strauss[48] and Landis and Hunt[49] show a difference between the fright (startle) reaction and the *Unklammerung* reflex described by Moro. According to Landis and Hunt, the startle reaction is originally a flexor reaction, while the Moro clasping reflex is an extensor reaction. Clarke[50] observed that the Moro reflex is the first to appear in the course of development. Later, some features of this reaction disappear, and extension becomes flexion as in the startle reaction. While Hunt[51] observed that both reactions can be elicited in the newborn during the course of normal development, as the Moro reflex is inhibited, the more mature startle/Strauss response takes over. Whereas both the withdrawal and Moro reflexes result in an immediate reaction to the stimulus, the Strauss reflex involves orientation to the stimulus followed by a conscious decision as to whether to react to it or simply ignore it as a non-threatening event. In other words, whereas the two more primitive reactions (freeze, fight or flight) result in immediate reaction *followed* by conscious awareness, the Strauss reflex involves arousal, orientation and cortical analysis *before* reaction.

Retention of primitive tonic neck and labyrinthine reflexes and/or under-developed head righting and associated protective equilibrium reactions (e.g. parachute reflex) can increase

---

*Parachute reflex develops in children in the second six months of life when you hold the child upright and then rotate his body quickly face forwards (as if falling). The baby will extend his/her arms forwards as if to break a fall, even though this reflex appears long before the baby walks. It provides a protective reaction during a fall and is linked to other righting reactions.

susceptibility to eliciting the Moro reflex when balance is destabilized, if there is a defect in one of the other sensory systems involved in orientation (e.g. vision or hearing) or as a result of psychological factors triggered by memory of similar events based on past experience. Individuals with a residual Moro reflex tend to be hyper-vigilant to any stimuli experienced as noxious in the past.

Myopia provides one example of a possible specific weakness in one sensory system resulting in increased vulnerability to a Moro reflex reaction under specific conditions. If corrective lenses are not worn and an object approaches at speed without prior warning, because the object cannot be seen until it is too close to catch or direct a defensive action, the visual stimulus can be sufficient to elicit the Moro reflex. In other words, the Moro reflex can act as, or is temporarily disinhibited as, a primitive defensive reaction under conditions where other 'higher' aspects of processing are not available. A similar reaction can be seen in patients who suffer from hyperacusis when exposed to certain frequencies of sound.

3.7 How to Use the INPP Screening Test

The INPP screening test for signs of Neuromotor Immaturity (NMI) in adults should *not* be used to form a diagnosis, but may be used to identify whether NMI is a factor in presenting symptoms of anxiety, panic disorder or agoraphobia, providing indications for more detailed medical investigations and treatment or referral for therapy aimed specifically at remediating signs of NMI in cooperation with psychological support.

It can be difficult to determine whether balance-related problems described by patients with psychological symptoms of anxiety, panic disorder and agoraphobia are caused by vestibular dysfunction or if the symptoms of vertigo originate from psychiatric disease. There can also be other physical factors involved including pathological factors (resulting from damage to specific areas in the CNS, mitral valve prolapse, low or high blood pressure, etc.) and endocrine factors (arising from rapid changes in hormone levels and thyroid function, hypoglycaemia or hypocalcaemia) or psychological factors, resulting from fear stemming from previous life events or as a secondary consequence of disorganized sensory processing. The possibility of underlying pathology should always be ruled out before referring adult patients for INPP therapy.

Simon et al. proposed three models to differentiate between organic and psychological factors:

1. **Psychosomatic model**: describes vestibular dysfunction as a consequence of anxiety. Hyperventilation and hyperarousal increase vestibulo-ocular reflex sensitivity, even among normals who hyperventilate. No studies have examined vestibular dysfunction during a panic attack.
2. **Somatopsychic model**: proposes that cases of panic disorder are triggered by misinterpreted internal stimuli (e.g. stimuli from vestibular dysfunction), that are interpreted as signifying imminent physical danger. Heightened sensitivity to vestibular sensations leads to increased anxiety and, through conditioning, drives the development of panic disorder.

3. **Network alarm theory**: derives from pharmacological challenge studies and other laboratory assessments of panic that suggest involvement of noradrenergic, serotonergic, and other connected neuronal systems. According to this theory, panic can be triggered by stimuli that set off a false alarm via afferents to the locus ceruleus, which then triggers the neuronal network. This network is thought to mediate anxiety and includes limbic, midbrain and prefrontal areas. Vestibular dysfunction in the setting of increased locus coeruleus sensitivity may be one potential trigger. The network alarm model contributes to a neuropsychiatric explanation for the somatopsychic model.[52]

Patients whose presenting symptoms fit the **somatopsychic** model, who *also* present with clear signs of neuromotor immaturity affecting the functioning of the vestibular system in the absence of pathology, are the ones most likely to benefit from rehabilitation training aimed directly at NMI. These patients also usually have a long-term history of difficulty in related areas stemming back to childhood.

All patients seen at INPP for assessment are first interviewed using the INPP Screening Questionnaire for Adults (Table 3.1).

Table 3.1

Adult screening questionnaire for neuromotor immaturity INPP

Name   Date of birth

Address

Tel No   Mobile No

Email

Has a diagnosis been given at any time ie. Dyslexia, Dyspraxia,
    ADHD, ADD, Agoraphobia, Panic Disorder or other?

If so, please state:

Are you currently taking any medication? Please list all:

Please list any existing medical conditions:

Have you at any time been treated for a psychiatric disorder? If
    so, please specify.

List your presenting symptoms:

3.8 The INPP Adult Screening Questionnaire

Part 1: Neurological development

Infancy

1. Is there any history of similar difficulties in your parents or their families? Yes/No
2. Were you conceived as a result of IVF? Yes/No
3. When your mother was pregnant with you, did she have any medical problems, for example, high blood pressure, excessive vomiting, threatened miscarriage, severe viral infection and severe emotional stress? Please state: Yes/No
   a. Did she smoke during pregnancy?
   b. Did she drink alcohol during pregnancy?
   c. Did she have a bad viral infection in the first 13 weeks?
   d. Was she under severe emotional stress between 25th and 27th week of her pregnancy?
   e. If known, how many ultra-sound scans were performed?
4. Were you born approximately at term, early for term or late for term? Yes/No
   Please give details
5. Was the birth process unusual or difficult in any way? Yes/No
   Induced (please state reason)
   Prolonged labour
   Precipitate (fast) labour
   Forceps
   Ventouse
   Caesarean section (elective or emergency)
   If yes, please give details
6. When you were born, were you small for term? Yes/No
   Please give birth weight, if known
7. When you were born, was there anything unusual about you, that is, the skull distorted, heavy bruising, definitely blue, heavily jaundiced, covered with a calcium-type coating or require intensive care? Yes/No
   If yes, please give details
8. In the first 13 weeks of your life, did you have difficulty in sucking, feeding or keeping food down? Yes/No
9. Were you breastfed? Yes/No
   How long did breastfeeding continue?
10. In the first 6 months of your life, were you a very still baby, so still that at times your mother wondered if it was a cot death? Yes/No
11. Between 6 months and 18 months, were you very active and demanding, requiring minimal sleep accompanied by continual screaming? Yes/No

12. When you were old enough to sit up in the pram and stand up in the cot, did you develop a violent rocking motion, so violent that either the pram or cot was actually moved? — Yes/No

13. Did you become a 'head-banger', that is, bang your head deliberately into solid objects? — Yes/No

14. Did you go through a motor stage of crawling on the stomach, followed by creeping on the hands and knees, or were you a 'bottom hopper' or 'roller' who one day stood up? — Yes/No
    If yes, please give details

15. Were you a child late at learning to walk? (later than 16 months) — Yes/No

16. Were you a child late at learning to talk? (two word phrases at two years, two to three word phrases at three years) — Yes/No

17. In the first 18 months of life, did you experience any illness involving high temperatures and/or convulsions? — Yes/No
    If yes, please give details

18. Was there any sign of infant eczema or asthma? — Yes/No
    Was there any sign of allergic responses? — Yes/No

19. Was there an adverse reaction to childhood vaccinations? — Yes/No

20. Did you have difficulty learning to dress? — Yes/No

21. Did you suck your thumb above the age of five years? — Yes/No
    If so, which thumb, right/left?

22. Did you wet the bed, albeit occasionally, above the age of five years? — Yes/No

23. Did you suffer from travel sickness? — Yes/No
    If so, at what age did travel sickness cease?
    Please specify which modes of transport elicit motion sickness

School

24. When you went to grade school, in the first two years of schooling, did you have problems learning to read? — Yes/No

25. In the first two years of formal schooling, did you have problems learning to write? — Yes/No

26. Did you have problems learning to do 'joined-up' or cursive writing? — Yes/No

27. Did you have difficulty learning to tell the time from a traditional clock face as opposed to a digital clock? — Yes/No

28. Did you have difficulty learning to ride a two-wheeled bicycle? — Yes/No

29. In the first eight years of your life, were you the child who continually suffered from colds, chest infections or ear problems? — Yes/No

30. Did you have difficulty in catching a ball, that is, eye–hand coordination problems? — Yes/No

31. When you were older and had to do gymnastics, did you have more trouble than all your classmates in doing things like forward rolls, handstands, climbing a rope, balancing or jumping over a vault horse? — Yes/No

32. Did you have difficulty sitting still, that is, had 'ants in the pants' and were continually being criticized by the teachers? — Yes/No

33. Did you make numerous mistakes when copying from a book or board? — Yes/No

34. When you wrote an essay or news item at school, did you occasionally put letters back to front or miss letters or words out? — Yes/No

Present: adulthood

35. If there is a sudden, unexpected noise or movement, do you over-react? — Yes/No

36. Do you have agoraphobia, panic attacks or extreme anxiety? — Yes/No
How old were you when these problems started?
What symptoms did you have?

37. Is there any one time or place where your symptoms are worse? — Yes/No
If yes, where or when?

38. Do you have feelings that at times you will fall over? — Often/Sometimes/Never

39. Do you see things moving which you know cannot move, that is, buildings, trees, etc.? — Often/Sometimes/Never

40. Do you ever feel that your eyes will not work properly at times, that is, that they do not focus properly or play tricks on you? — Often/Sometimes/Never

41. Do you suffer from feelings of nausea? — Often/Sometimes/Never

42. Do you have feelings of dizziness? — Often/Sometimes/Never

43. Do you have feelings of dizziness while lying in bed? — Often/Sometimes/Never

44. Do you feel that you have poor balance? — Yes/No

45. Do you feel your coordination is very bad at times? — Yes/No

Part 3

46. Do you suffer or have you suffered from migraine? — Often/Sometimes/Never

47. Are you very sensitive to bright lights? — Yes/No
(Have you been to a discotheque with flashing lights, and does this affect you?)

48. Would you say that you are more sensitive to sound than everyone you know? — Yes/No

49. Do you have problems in sorting out which is left and right when giving directions or sorting out which is your left and right hand? — Yes/No

50. When you are writing something long and complicated, do you find that after a time you begin to make silly mistakes, such as putting letters in the wrong order or words in the wrong order, or your ability to spell even simple words becomes difficult?

Often/Sometimes/Never

51. When you are very, very tired, do you find that you know what you want to say but what you do say actually comes out jumbled up?

Often/Sometimes/Never

52. When you are very, very tired, do you find that your coordination goes and you bump into things or become clumsy?

Often/Sometimes/Never

Please add any extra information you think may be appropriate.

3.9 Interpreting the INPP Adult Screening Questionnaire

Adults for whom the INPP method is appropriate have a history of a *cluster* of small issues relating to balance, coordination and visual perception from childhood, for which they were able to compensate reasonably well until either the onset of puberty, early adult life or a precipitating event in adult life. Individuals with anxiety and NMI typically have a history which includes at least seven of the following:

- Illnesses involving very high temperatures with or without febrile convulsions in childhood
- Unable to perform forward rolls, vault over a horse, etc. in physical education classes at school
- Dislike or avoidance of playground equipment, which involves vestibular stimulation (swings, whirligigs, seesaws etc.)
- Motion sickness *which continued beyond puberty*
- Migraines which started from puberty
- Feelings of that they might fall over
- Momentary optical illusions
- Feeling of nausea
- Feelings of dizziness, sometimes when lying in bed
- Awareness of poor balance
- Poor coordination
- Sensitivity to bright lights
- Sensitivity to sound
- Difficulty sorting out left and right

Additionally, adults who *also* present with a history of specific learning difficulties may report:

- History of repeated ear, nose or throat infections in childhood.
- When writing something long and complicated, after a time they begin to make mistakes such as putting letters in the wrong order or their ability to spell simple words deteriorates.
- When tired, speech and coordination become jumbled and confused.

However, specific learning difficulties are not necessarily present in this adult population. Many have demonstrated educational ability and achievement to tertiary level and only start to produce symptoms of anxiety when placed under examination conditions or occupational, hormonal or emotional stress, consistent with Blythe's theory of previous compensation.

In using the questionnaire as a screening instrument, a score greater than 7 'yes' answers on the *numbered* questions provides an indication that NMI might underlie some of the presenting symptoms and that further tests to confirm or eliminate the possibility are warranted.

The answers are scored:

   0. 'No' or 'never' answer
   1. 'Yes' or 'often' answer
   2. ½ for 'sometimes' answer

Only one point is allocated for each numbered question irrespective of whether the patient has ticked several factors listed as sub-questions. For example, under question 5,

"Was the birth process unusual or difficult in any way?" A score of 1 will be given even if the patient has ticked indicating that any of the following occurred: (i) labour was induced, (ii) labour was prolonged and (iii) forceps were used.

It is recommended that when investigating the possibility of NMI in adults, the screening questionnaire is used prior to the screening tests.

The INPP method is *not* recommended to treat patients with psychiatric illness or with a history of psychiatric illness (e.g. schizophrenia, psychosis, bipolar disorder).

It should also be noted that adults with a long history of NMI can find it difficult to make the behavioural adjustments needed as their profile changes and may need counselling support to help them through the emotional process of adaptation. For this reason, INPP recommends independent counselling and that practitioners working with the INPP method with adults presenting with anxiety, agoraphobia or panic disorder have an additional qualification in psychology.

References

1   Blythe, P (1979) Personal communication.

2   Hain, TC and Helminski, JO (2007) Anatomy and physiology of the normal vestibular system. In: Herdman, SJ (ed.), *Vestibular rehabilitation*, 3rd edn. F.A. Davis Company, Philadelphia, PA. pp. 2–18.

3   Berthoz, A (2012) *Simplexity: simplifying principles for a complex world.* Yale University Press, New Haven, CT.

4   Manali, SA and Meyers, AD. (2012 February 24) Vestibular Reflex Testing. http://emedicine. medscape.com/article/1836134-overview. Accessed February 14, 2013.

5   Kandel, ER, Schwartz, JK and Jessell, TM (1991) *The principles of neuroscience.* Elsevier Publishing Co. Inc., New York.

6   Blythe, P (1990) Panic disorder and its non-neurotic causation. Paper presented at the INPP International Conference Guernsey CI. September 1990.

7   Cohen, BH (2009) The neural substrate of the subjective experience of anxiety. Poster presented at the annual meeting of the Social and Affective Neuroscience Society, New York University, New York. October 2009.

8   Cox, JM (1804) *Practical observations in insanity*. Baldwin and Murray, London. p. 106.

9   Benedikt, M (1870) Über Platzschwindel. *Aligemeine Wiener Medizinische Zeitung*, **15**: 488.

10 Lannois, M and Tournier, C (1899). Les lesions auriculaires sont une cause déterminante fréquente de l'agoraphobie. *Annals des maladies de l'oreille due larynx, du nez, et du pharynx*, **14**: 286-301.

11 Bauer, J (1916) Der Baranusche Zeigeveruch etc. bie traumatischen neurosen. *Wiener Klinisch Wochenschrift*: 40.

12 Leidler, R and Loewy, K (1923) Der Swindel der Neurosen. *Monatsschrift für Ohrenheilkunde und Laryngo Rhinologie*, **57**(1).

13 Schilder, PH (1933) The vestibular apparatus in neurosis and psychosis. *Journal of Nervous and Mental Disease*, **78**(1-23): 137-164.

14 Von Weizsäcker, V Cited in Paul Schilder (1933). The vestibular apparatus in neurosis and psychosis. *Journal of Nervous and Mental Disease*, **78**: 1-23.

15 Goldstein, Cited in Paul Schilder (1933). The vestibular apparatus in neurosis and psychosis. *Journal of Nervous and Mental Disease*, **78**: 1-23.

16 Frank, J and Levinson, HN (1976-1977) Seasickness mechanisms and medications in dysmetric dyslexia and dyspraxia. *Academic Therapy*, **12**: 1-24.

17 Frank, J and Levinson, HN (1977) Antimotion sickness medications in dysmetric dyslexia and dyspraxia. *Academic Therapy*, **12**: 411-425.

18 Levinson, HN (1980) *A solution to the riddle dyslexia*. Springer-Verlag, New York.

19 Levinson, HN (1984) *Smart but feeling dumb*. Warner, New York.

20 Levinson, HN (1986) *Phobia free*. Evans, New York.

21 Reason, JT and Brand, JJ (1975) *Motion sickness*. Academic Press, London.

22 Brand, JJ and Perry, WLM (1966). Drugs used in motion sickness. *Pharmacological Reviews*, **18**: 895-924.

23 De Quirós, JB, and Schrager, OL (1978) *Neurological fundamentals in learning disabilities*. Academic Therapy Publications Inc., Novato, CA.

24 Blythe, P and McGlown, DJ (1979) *An organic basis for neuroses and educational difficulties*. Insight Publications, Chester.

25 Selye, H (1974) In: Gunderson, EKE and Rahe, RH (eds), *Life stress and illness*. Charles C Thomas, Springfield, IL.

26 Le Winn, E (1969) *Human neurological organisation*. Charles C Thomas, Springfield, IL.

27 Blythe, P and McGlown, DJ (1982 July) Agoraphobia - is it organic? *World Medicine*, **1982**: 57-59.

28 Levinson, HN (1989 February) The cerebellar-vestibular predisposition to anxiety disorders. *Perceptual & Motor Skills*, **68**(1): 323-338.

29 Carr, DB and Sheehan, DV (1984) Evidence that panic disorder has a metabolic cause. In: Ballenger, JC (ed.), *Biology of agoraphobia*. American Psychiatric Press, Washington, DC. pp. 100-111.

30 Redmond, DE (1977) Alterations in the function of the nucleus locus coeruleus: a possible model for studies in anxiety. In Hanin, I and Usdin, E (eds.), *Animal models in psychiatry and neurology*. Pergamon, New York. pp. 293-304.

31 Redmond, DE and Huang, YH (1979) New evidence for a locus coeruleus-norepinephrine connection with anxiety. *Life Science*, **25**(26): 2149-2162.

32 Forrest, DS (2002) Prevalence of primitive reflexes in patients with anxiety disorders. Thesis submitted to the University of Edinburgh in part fulfilment of Doctorate in Clinical Psychology.

33 Yardley, L and Redfern, MS (2001) Psychological factors influencing recovery from balance disorders. *Journal of Anxiety Disorders*, **15**(1-2): 107-119.

34 Nardi, AE, Lopes, FL, Valenca, AM, Nascimento, I, Mezzasalma, MA and Zin, WA (2004) Psychopathological description of hyperventilation-induced panic attacks: a comparison with spontaneous panic attacks. *Psychopathology*, **37**(1): 29–35.

35 Sakellari, V, Bronstein, AM, Corna, S, Hammon, CA, Jones, S and Wolsley, CJ (1997) The effects of hyperventilation on postural control mechanisms. *Brain*, **120**(9): 1659–1673.

36 Minor, LB, Haslwanter, T, Straumann, D and Zee, DS (1999) Hyperventilation-induced nystagmus in patients with vestibular schwannoma. *Neurology*, **53**(9): 2158–2168.

37 Holmberg, J (2006) *Dizziness and fear of falling: a behavioural and physiological approach to 'Phobic Postural Vertigo,'* University of Lund, Lund.

38 Yardley, L, Luxon, L and Lear, S (1994) Vestibular and posturographic test results in people with symptoms of panic and agoraphobia. *Journal of Audiological Medicine*, **3**: 48–65.

39 Jacob, RG, Moller, MB, Turner, SM and Wall, C (1985) Otoneurological examination in panic disorder and agoraphobia with panic attacks: a pilot study. *The American Journal of Psychiatry*, **142**(6): 715–720.

40 Jacob, RG, Furman, JM, Durrant, JD and Turner, SM (1997) Surface dependence: a balance control strategy in panic disorder with agoraphobia. *Psychosomatic Medicine*, **59**(3): 323–330.

41 Jacob, RG, Redfern, MS and Furman, JM (1995) Optic flow-induced sway in anxiety disorder with space and motion discomfort. *Journal of Anxiety Disorders*, **9**(5): 411–425.

42 Bein-Wierzbinski, W (2001). Persistent primitive reflexes in elementary school children. Effect on oculomotor and visual perception. Paper presented at the 13th European Conference of Neuro-developmental Delay in Children with Specific Learning Difficulties. Chester, UK. March 2001.

43 Wilson, VJ, Boyle, R, Fukushima, K, Rose, PK, Shinoda, Y, Sugiuchi,Y and Uchino, Y (1995) The vestibulocollic reflex. *Journal of Vestibular Research*, **5**(3): 147–170.

44 Hain, TC (2009). Postural, vestibulospinal and vestibulocollic reflexes. http://www.dizziness-and-balance.com/anatomy/vspine.htm. Accessed January 17, 2014.

45 Welgampola, MS and Colebatch, JG (2001 November) Vestibulocollic reflexes: normal values and the effect of age. *Clinical Neurophysiology*, **112**(11): 1971–1979.

46 Jacobs, RJ (1979) Visual resolution and contour interaction in the fovea and periphery. *Vision Research*, **19**(11): 1187–1195.

47 Carpenter, RH, Cronly-Dillon, JR and Leventhal, AG (1991) *Eye Movements: Vision and Visual Dysfunction Series*. Vol 8. CRC Press, Boca Raton, FL. pp. 1–10.

48 Strauss, H (1929) Das zusammenschrecken. *Journal für Psychologie und Neurologie*, **39**: 111.

49 Landis, C and Hunt, WA (1963) The startle pattern. Cited in Peiper A. (ed.), *Cerebral function in infancy and childhood*. Consultants Bureau, New York.

50 Clarke, FM (1939) A developmental study of the bodily reactions of infants to an auditory stimulus. *Journal of Genetic Psychology*, **55**: 415–427.

51 Hunt, WA (1939) 'Body jerk' as a concept describing infant behavior. *Journal of Genetic Psychology*, **55**: 215–220.

52 Simon, NM, Pollack, MH, Tuby, KS and Stern, TA (1998) Dizziness and panic disorder: a review of the association between vestibular dysfunction and anxiety. *Annals of Clinical Psychiatry*, **10**: 75–80.

4

INPP Screening Test for Signs of Neuromotor Immaturity in Adults

4.1 General Instructions

Testing should be carried out with the test subject wearing loose clothing and in bare feet on firm, level ground.

For timed tests (Romberg and advanced Romberg), a stopwatch with a second hand should be used.

To ensure that the test subject has understood verbal instructions correctly, the tester should also demonstrate the beginning of each test procedure.

Additional notes of observations made during tests should be recorded on the separate observation sheets provided and attached to the final score sheet. These observations provide additional information about qualitative performance and may be referred to before and after intervention.

4.2 Scoring

All tests are scored using a five-point rating scale:

0. No Abnormality Detected (NAD)
1. 25% dysfunction
2. 50% dysfunction
3. 75% dysfunction
4. 100% dysfunction

4.3 Screening Tests for Use with Adults

- Romberg test
- Mann test (advanced Romberg test)
- Tandem walk

- Fog walk
- Quadruped test for the ATNR (Ayres 1 test)
- Hoff–Schilder test for the ATNR
- Quadruped test for the STNR
- Erect test for the TLR
- Standard test for the Moro reflex
- Erect test for the Moro reflex (drag back test)

4.4 Tests for Balance and 'Soft Signs' of Neurological Dysfunction (ND)

Tests for balance, proprioception and postural stability and static balance (Romberg and Mann tests) and tests for soft signs of Neurological Dysfunction (ND) and dynamic balance (Tandem and Fog walks) can be used to provide indications of neurological dysfunction. These tests are not specific for the vestibular-spinal system but simply provide information regarding postural stability.

Because balance is maintained through the integration at the brainstem level of information from the vestibular end organs and the visual and proprioceptive sensory modalities – this processing takes place in the vestibular nuclei, with modulating influences from higher centres including the cerebellum, the extrapyramidal system, the cerebral cortex and the contiguous reticular formation – any derangement of the structure or function of the sensory inputs, the central vestibular structures or the effector pathways (the oculo-motor and vestibular–spinal pathways) is likely to result in a balance disorder. These may occur as a result of primary pathology (refer for further medical investigations, diagnosis and treatment) or be secondary symptoms of underlying Neurological Dysfunction (ND).[1] This *second* group may benefit from various remedial interventions including the INPP programme.

Similarly, it should be borne in mind that general medical conditions can contribute to dizziness. These include but are not exclusive to postural hypotension, vasovagal syncope, cardiac valvular disease, hyperventilation, specific skeletal problems and others. It is therefore vital that a full and comprehensive history is taken and such causal factors are eliminated or taken into account before using the screening test for NMI. A general medical examination, with particular attention to the eyes, the ears, the nervous system, the cardiovascular system and the locomotor system, may be indicated, and general medical investigations should also be considered prior to using the screening test.

The Tandem and Fog walks are tests for 'soft signs' of neurological dysfunction. Neurological Soft Signs (NSS) are minor ('soft') neurological abnormalities in sensory and motor performance identified by clinical examination. There is still a lack of consensus on the neuro-dysfunctional area underlying NSS; some authors suggest that NSS reflect a failure in the integration within or between sensory and motor systems,[2] whereas others advocate deficits in neuronal circuits involving subcortical structures (e.g. basal ganglia, brainstem and limbic system).[3] While NSS do not isolate the aetiology of the presenting signs, they can provide useful markers of NMI as a significant underlying factor and additional measures with which to evaluate change during or following intervention.

Age should also be taken into account when using the Romberg and Mann tests and the Tandem and Fog walks:

> Advanced age is a risk factor because vestibular ganglion cell counts decrease with age. By the time someone has reached 80 years of age, only about 50% of vestibular neurons still remain. This reduction presumably contributes to the invariable loss of balance function that occurs as people age. Multi-sensory dizziness, particularly in the elderly, can occur when two or more of the following conditions are present: visual impairment, peripheral neuropathy, vestibular deficit, cervical spondylosis, and orthopaedic disorders affecting the large joints. An appreciation that disequilibrium may be consequent on multiple pathologies is essential if the appropriate investigation and interpretation of the data are to be achieved.[2]

A study carried out in 2011 that investigated normative data for the modified Romberg test in adults in the United States found that the length of time a person can maintain balance on the Romberg test starts to decline gradually from 30 seconds between 40 and 49 years of age and in general the threshold of 20 seconds is crossed between 60 and 69 years of age. Subjects of 80+ years could only maintain balance for up to 9 seconds.[4] These general parameters should be taken into account when using the Romberg and Mann tests.

4.5 Tests for Balance and Proprioception

The Romberg test

The Romberg test examines posterior column function and when used as part of a neurological examination can only be administered if the patient is able to stand steadily with the eyes open when the test is used. Under these conditions, the Romberg test does not test the ability to stand, but to maintain posture without visual input, which requires proprioception. Under these test conditions, the Romberg sign is 'positive' if the patient can maintain balance with the eyes open but falls when the eyes are closed.

INPP applies the Romberg and Mann tests in a broader context to evaluate control of standing balance, proprioception and subjective experience of dizziness or anxiety while performing the tests. Equal attention is paid to control of balance, degree of sway, synkinesia and subjective experience of disorientation with the eyes open and closed.

Further isolation of sensory cues under conditions which stress balance can be included in more detailed diagnostic assessments such as repeating the Romberg and Mann tests under conditions with a decreased base of support (e.g. standing on soft foam rubber), which distort proprioceptive feedback.

Test procedure: Romberg test

Test position

Standing up straight, feet together, arms and hands to the side and looking straight ahead (Figure 4.1a). *Assessor should stand behind the test subject* ready to catch in case there is a loss of balance.

Eyes open

The test subject is instructed to stand still and continue looking straight ahead.

This position should be maintained for approximately 30+ seconds (unless age or other medical conditions indicate a shorter duration[4]).

Eyes closed

He or she is then asked to maintain the position but to close the eyes and 'imagine' – pretend – that he/she is looking straight ahead. Hold the position for 30+ seconds or age-appropriate time (Figure 4.1b).

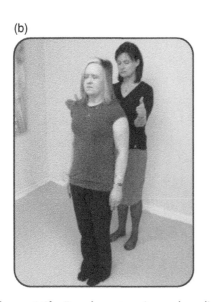

(a)

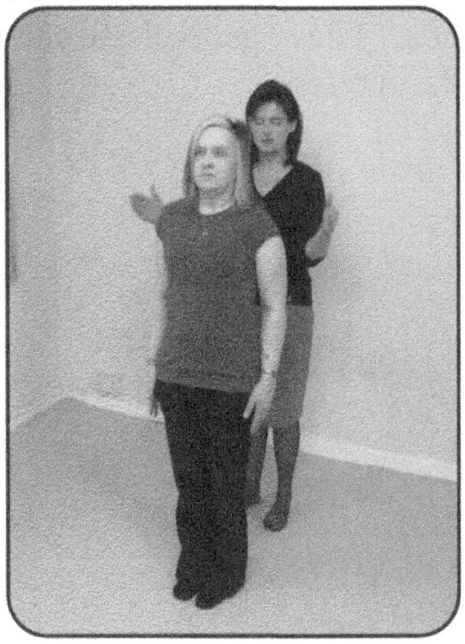

Figure 4.1a Romberg test (eyes open).

(b)

Figure 4.1b Romberg test (eyes closed).

Observations

Eyes open (qualitative observations)

- Time the number of seconds the patient can maintain balance without moving their feet from the proper position.
- Is there noticeable sway?
- If so, in which direction – backwards, forwards, to the left or right side or in a circular movement?
- How much does he/she sway?
- Do one or both arms move out and away from the body?
- Does the face become contorted?
- Is there loss of balance?
- Is there a marked increase in anxiety after closing the eyes?
- What is the test subject's *subjective* experience during the test?

Clinical observations of adult patients assessed by INPP practitioners have shown that observations of the Romberg and subsequent Mann tests alone are not the best indicators of Neuromotor Dysfunction (NMD) in patients presenting with symptoms of agoraphobia and/or panic disorder:

> The most accurate indicator of vestibular or vestibular-proprioceptive disturbance in these comes from observation of problems with balance *and* the patient's *subjective* experience of undertaking the test procedures, obtained by asking the test subject to demonstrate with their fingers how much they feel like they are moving during the Romberg and Mann tests. Most commonly they overestimate from two to five times the distance observed. Although little or no sway may be observed, to the patient it feels like much more. This can provide an indication of the degree of cortical effort employed in compensating for the underlying dysfunction.
>
> Conversely, a patient may exhibit a significant sway, but feel little or no movement. These patients are the ones that consistently feel a compulsion to move. If their movement is restricted, they begin to feel anxious. Empirical evidence based on clinical observations indicate that stimulant medications do not work in these cases.[5]

Eyes closed

Note all of the observations listed under the section 'The Romberg test' for scoring with eyes open, paying particular attention to the degree of difficulty outlined.

If the patient was able to maintain control of balance with the eyes open but loses control when the eyes are closed, the Romberg test is described as 'positive', indicating problems with proprioception or vestibular functioning.

If the patient is able to maintain the position for the required time with the eyes open but balance is unstable and there is a marked increase in instability when the eyes are closed, this might indicate vestibular dysfunction.

If balance is impaired with the eyes open, there may be a problem with the cerebellum, but the Romberg test should not be used in isolation as an indicator of cerebellar involvement.

The following conditions may also elicit a positive result on the Romberg test:

- Vitamin B12 deficiency
- Conditions affecting the dorsal columns of the spinal cord such as tabes dorsalis
- Conditions affecting the sensory nerves such as diabetic peripheral large-fibre neuropathy
- Friedreich's ataxia

Scoring

Eyes open

0. None of the observations are noted.
1. Slight sway in any direction, slight movement of the arms away from the sides of the body and slight face or tongue involvement.
2. More marked sway, more marked movement of the arms away from the body and a more marked facial or tongue involvement.
3. Near loss of balance and need to extend the arms in a 'primary balance' position to maintain balance.
4. Loss of balance.

Also note the patient's subjective experience of the test procedure by asking them either to indicate with the fingers of both hands how unsteady they feel or to say on a scale of 0–10 (0 = NAD and 10 = loss of balance) how unsteady they felt.

Eyes closed

0. None of the observations are noted.
1. Slight sway in any direction, slight movement of the arms away from the sides of the body and slight face or tongue involvement.
2. More marked sway, more marked movement of the arms away from the body and a more marked facial or tongue involvement.
3. Near loss of balance and need to extend the arms in a 'primary balance' position to maintain balance.
4. Loss of balance.

Also note the patient's subjective experience of the test procedure by asking them either to indicate with the fingers of both hands how unsteady they feel or to say on a scale of 0–10 (0 = NAD and 10 = loss of balance) how unsteady they felt. Record this information on the observation sheet.

The Mann test (advanced Romberg test)

This test is also sometimes referred to as the Sharpened Romberg (SR) or Tandem Romberg. The test provides an additional measure of balance and equilibrium over a narrowed base of support and requires a higher level of skill than the Romberg test.

The advanced Romberg test is carried out in a standing position with one foot placed in front of the other at the midline, heel touching the toe. For screening purposes, the test subject is not instructed which foot to place in front. The screening test simply observes which foot is selected. (The test may be repeated swapping the foot position.)

Age norms for time on this test vary. Some sources stipulate 60 seconds with the eyes open and closed[6]; others only 10 seconds.[7-9] Some decrease in time is expected in adults after 60 years of age, with deterioration likely to advance with age thereafter. For screening purposes, INPP recommends up to 30 seconds in adolescents over the age of 16 and adults or for as long as they are able within a 30 second period. Subjects are allowed one trial test before evaluation.

Timing is stopped if subjects move their feet from the proper position, if they open their eyes on eyes-closed trials or if they reach their maximum balance times of 30 seconds.

(a)

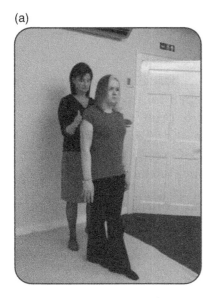

Figure 4.2a Test position for the Mann test (eyes open).

Test procedure: Mann test (advanced Romberg test), eyes open

Test position

Stand with one foot placed in front of the other, with heel touching the toe and the arms down by the sides (Figure 4.2a).

Instruction

Stand still with one foot placed directly in front of the other, heel touching the toe (also demonstrate). *Maintain this position, if you can, for up to 30 seconds.*

Observations

- Can the patient adapt from the Romberg test position to the heel–toe position with required alteration in weight distribution?
- Is there any difficulty in bringing the foot to the midline or maintaining balance at the midline?
- Do the arms become involved in maintaining balance?
- Is there marked sway or unsteadiness? If so, after how many seconds and in which direction(s)?
- Is there involvement of other parts of the body in continuous movements in the attempt to maintain balance?

- If they 'feel' unstable, but there is no visible evidence of instability (subjective), it may suggest vestibular–proprioceptive mismatch.

Scoring

0. None of the observations are noted (NAD).
1. Slight difficulty in adjusting to altered plane of reference observed in sway in any direction, slight movement of the arms away from the sides of the body and slight face or tongue involvement.
2. More marked sway, more marked movement of the arms away from the body and more marked facial or tongue involvement.
3. Near loss of balance, need to extend the arms in a 'primary balance' position to maintain balance and constant motion.
4. Loss of balance.

(b)

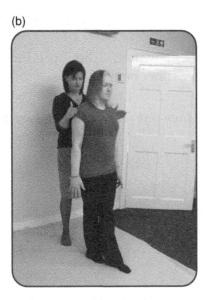

Figure 4.2b Test position for the Mann test (eyes closed).

Test procedure: Mann test (advanced Romberg), eyes closed

Test position

After 30 seconds, instruct the test subject to maintain the position and to close the eyes (Figure 4.2b).

If the test subject has failed to maintain balance with the eyes open for up to 30 seconds, allow them to have a brief rest, assume the test position again and then close the eyes. Time the number of seconds the patient can maintain balance with the eyes closed.

Test subjects are permitted one trial run with the eyes open and closed.

Observations

Is there a marked increase in any of the aforementioned observations when the eyes are closed?

Scoring

0. None of the observations are noted (NAD).
1. Slight difficulty maintaining balance observed in sway, slight movement of the arms away from the sides of the body and slight face or tongue involvement.
2. More marked sway, more marked movement of the arms away from the body and more marked facial or tongue involvement.
3. Near loss of balance, need to extend the arms in a 'primary balance' position to maintain balance and constant motion.
4. Loss of balance.

The Tandem walk

The Tandem walk is used primarily to assess balance, gait and signs of possible cerebellar involvement.

Patients with *truncal ataxia* caused by damage to the cerebellar vermis or associated pathways will have particular difficulty with this task, since they tend to have a wide-based, unsteady gait and become more unsteady when attempting to keep their feet close together.

Both the Tandem walk and walking on the outsides of the feet (Fog walk) are performed forwards and backwards. When going forwards, the primary sensory system involved in coordination is vision; when going backwards, balance and proprioception take over the leading roles. If a person's performance is *consistently and significantly* better on *both* tests in one direction only, it might indicate:

a) Forwards consistently better than backwards – vision is being used to compensate for difficulties with balance and/or proprioception.
b) Backwards consistently better than forwards – the primary dysfunctional system may be the visual system.

Test procedure: The Tandem walk

Test position: standing and the eyes open

Instruct the test subject to walk *slowly* in a straight line with the heel of the leading foot making contact with the toes of the trailing foot each time the leading foot is placed on the ground:

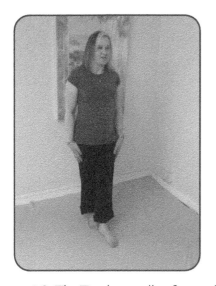

Figure 4.3 The Tandem walk – forwards.

1. Forwards (Figure 4.3)
2. Backwards (the toe of the leading foot making contact with the heel of the trailing foot and then the leading foot is placed on the ground)

Score separately for forwards and backwards.

Observations

General: Note any problems with balance, coordination and position of the limbs:

- Observe control of balance. Is there marked difficulty in maintaining balance?
- Is there difficulty in:

1. Placing the foot at the midline (may indicate cerebellar involvement)
2. Maintaining balance when the feet are positioned at the midline

- Does the patient need to hold the arms out in a primary balance position or use excessive arm movements in order to complete the test (indicative of need to widen frame of reference to compensate for difficulty with maintaining balance over a narrow base of support)?
- Check accuracy of foot placement (proprioceptive awareness).
- Note degree of difficulty/concentration used to carry out the task.
- Note any 'overflow' of movement, for example, facial, mouth or tongue involvement.
- Note the speed at which the test is performed. If too fast, remind the subject once to slow down. If the subject can only maintain control when moving fast and any of the aforementioned signs emerge when movement is slowed down, it might indicate a tendency to use speed to compensate for poor control of balance.

Scoring

Record *separate* scores for performance forwards and backwards using the following scale:

0. NAD
1. Minimal problems noted with the following: balance or foot placement, tendency to fixate visually on one point, slight facial involvement, tendency to look down at the feet and slight hand or arm involvement
2. Increase in any or several of the aforementioned observations, use of 'primary balance' position, some difficulty in controlling balance at the midline and test performed too fast
3. Near loss of balance, arms extended, sway in the arms and/or body and inaccuracy in foot placement
4. Loss of balance with or without marked increase in any of the aforementioned observations and inability to place the foot at the midline

The Fog walk (1963[10]) (walking on the outsides of the feet)

It is a test primarily used in medicine to elicit vertical synkinesia.

The patient is instructed to walk slowly in a straight line for a distance of 3–4 metres on the outsides of the feet keeping the arms to the sides.

Going on to the outsides of the feet can elicit abnormal posturing and/or associated movements of the upper extremities. Associated movements are defined as movements that accompany a motor function, are not involved in the specific motor function and are not necessary to its performance. The persistence of associated movements is a sign supporting other evidence of immaturity in the brain or of poor development of discriminatory, selective motor activity.[11]

Test procedure

Test position: standing and eyes open

Instruct the test subject to walk *slowly* in a straight line on the outsides of the feet for a distance of approximately 4 metres: (a) forwards (Figure 4.4a) and (b) backwards (Figure 4.4b).

(a) 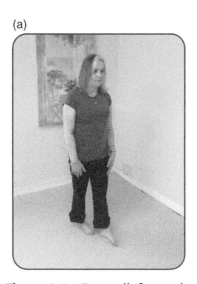 (b)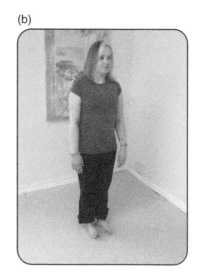

Figure 4.4a Fog walk forwards.   **Figure 4.4b** Fog walk backwards.

After completing the distance forwards, instruct the subject to stop, put the feet together and stand still and then to repeat the procedure going backwards. Score separately for forwards and backwards.

Observations

- Note any difficulty staying on the outside of the feet (e.g. tendency to walk on the heels).
- Alteration in posture/mild vertical synkinesia.
- Coordination.

- Position of the hands or arms such as partial rotation of both hands or gripping (cupping), hemiplegia or palmar grasp.
- Movements of the mouth.

Scoring

Record *separate* scores for performance forwards and backwards using the following scale:

0. NAD
1. Slight involuntary hand involvement on one side
2. Hand involvement on both sides and/or slight postural alteration or not fully on the outsides of the feet and/or facial involvement
3. Simian posture, stiff gait with homolateral movements or marked hemiplegia
4. Marked simian posture and unable to move or complete the task

4.6 Tests for Primitive Reflexes

Asymmetrical Tonic Neck Reflex (ATNR)

There are a variety of tests available to test for the continued presence of the ATNR. In young babies, the reflex is assessed in the supine position with the tester gently rotating the head to each side. Head rotation elicits extension of the limbs on the jaw side and flexion of the occipital limbs up to six months of age.

The supine test is suitable for use with very young children or individuals with physical handicap who are unable to maintain either the quadruped or erect postures. However, as muscle tone develops, the ATNR can be 'masked' by alteration in the general level of muscle tension present during testing, and for this reason, the supine test is not included in the screening test for adults. More sensitive tests for eliciting the ATNR in adults include the quadruped test[11] and the Hoff–Schilder test.[12]

In the quadruped test, the test subject is instructed to go on hands and knees in a 'table' position (Figure 4.5a) with the back of the head held level with the spine. The tester gently rotates the head as far as possible to one side (Figure 4.5b). If the ATNR is present as the head is turned, flexion will occur in the *occipital* arm. There may also be some flexion of the hip on the occipital side. The reflex may be present on one side only or vary in strength on either side. The tester observes the degree of flexion in the occipital arm when the head is turned to each side.

The ATNR is scored in the direction to which the head is turned. That is, when the head is turned to the right, the tester will observe the degree of flexion in the *left* occipital arm; if flexion is observed on the occipital side, the tester will record the degree of flexion as evidence of the ATNR being present to the *right*.

Ayres quadruped test for the ATNR[11]

Test procedure

Test position: hands and knees

Instruct the child to go on hands and knees into the 'table' or four-point kneeling position (Figure 4.5a):

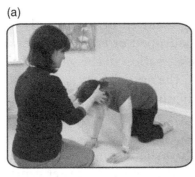 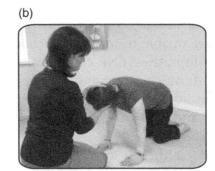

(a)   (b)

Figure 4.5a Ayres test position.   **Figure 4.5b** Ayres test – head rotation.

- The tester kneels in front of the subject and slowly rotates his/her head to one side, keeping the head parallel to the shoulder line (Figure 4.5b); when rotated, pause in this position for 5–10 seconds.
- Return the head to the midline; pause for 5–10 seconds.
- Turn the head to the opposite side; pause for 5–10 seconds.
- Return to the midline; pause for 5–10 seconds.
- Repeat the sequence four times. If the result is markedly positive on the first or second rotation, it is not necessary to repeat the procedure four times.

Observations

- As the subject's head is turned to one side, does the occipital arm or shoulder bend at the elbow, or is there any flexion at the hip on the occipital side?

Score the reflex as being on the side to which the head is turned.

Scoring

0. No movement of the opposite arm, shoulder or hip (**reflex not present**).
1. Slight bending of the opposite arm or movement of the shoulder or hip (**reflex present up to 25%**).
2. Definite bending of the opposite arm or movement of the shoulder or hip (**reflex present up to 50%**).
   Marked bending of the opposite arm, with or without shoulder or hip involvement (**reflex present up to 75%**).
   Collapse of the occipital arm as a result of head rotation. There may also be hip involvement (**reflex 100% retained**).

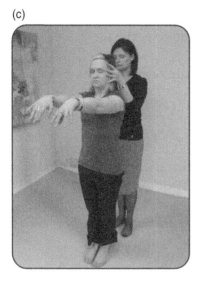

Figure 4.5c Test position for the Hoff–Schilder test.

Asymmetrical Tonic Neck Reflex adapted Hoff–Schilder (erect) test

Test procedure

Test position

Erect, feet together, arms extended at shoulder height to the front, wrists flexed and hands relaxed* and eyes closed. Tester stands behind the test subject (Figure 4.5c).

The subject is instructed as follows: 'Stand with your feet together, arms stretched out at shoulder height and wrists floppy. Close your eyes. I am going to turn your head to each side, but I want your arms to remain where they are.'

Demonstrate the first part of the test procedure:

- Slowly rotate the head to one side (Figure 4.5d).
- Pause for 5–10 seconds.
- Slowly return the head to the midline.
- Pause for 5–10 seconds.
- Slowly rotate the head to the other side (Figure 4.5e).

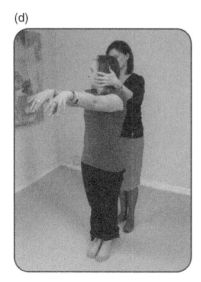

Figure 4.5d Hoff Schilder Test – Head rotation to the right.

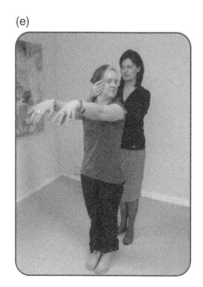

Figure 4.5e Hoff Schilder Test – Head rotation to the left.

*The original Hoff–Schilder test does not instruct the patient to flex the wrists. INPP has added this to the test, as some test subjects extend the hands before testing, enabling them to control the degree of movement in the arms when the head is rotated, obscuring the true extent of reflex present.

- Repeat the sequence 2–3 times.
- Repeat once more, turning the head quickly (but carefully) to each side.

If there is any pain or resistance on head rotation, do *not* continue to rotate the head beyond this point.

Observations

- Note any movement of the arm(s) in the direction of head rotation or counter-movement of the hips. (The latter might indicate retention of the ATNR in the legs.)
- Note any gravitational insecurity as a result of closing the eyes on head rotation.
- Is the balance affected? This can be as a result of vestibular stimulation and/or ATNR in the legs.

Scoring

0. No movement of the arms in response to head rotation
1. Slight rotation of the arm(s) in the direction of head rotation up to 12–15°
2. Rotation of the arms up to 30°
3. Rotation of the arms up to 45°
4. 90° rotation of the arms

The Symmetrical Tonic Neck Reflex (STNR)

In the infant, flexion of the head in the quadruped position will elicit bending of the arms and extension of the legs; extension of the head in the quadruped position will elicit extension in the arms and flexion in the legs.

The test subject is instructed to go on hands and knees in the 'table' position and to look upwards 'as if looking towards the ceiling', arching the head (not the back) upwards and backwards. If the reflex is present in extension as the head is lifted, the legs bend, either pulling the buttocks towards the heels or the heels towards the buttocks, and the arms straighten.

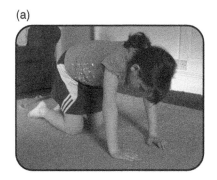

Figure 4.6a STNR quadruped test position.

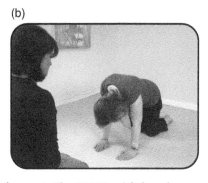

Figure 4.6b STNR with head flexion.

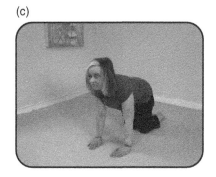

Figure 4.6c STNR with head extension.

The test subject is then instructed to look down 'as if looking between your knees'. If the reflex is present in flexion as the head is flexed, the arms will bend and there may also be elevation of the feet.

Test procedure

Test position: hands and knees

- Instruct the test subject to go on hands and knees in the four-point kneeling 'table' position (Figure 4.6a).
- The patient is instructed to maintain the test position in the arms and the legs and to slowly bend the head down 'as if looking between your knees while keeping your arms straight and the remainder of your body still' (Figure 4.6b).
- Hold the position for five seconds and then slowly move the head upwards 'as if looking at the ceiling' (Figure 4.6c). Repeat up to six times.

Observations

- Note any bending of the arms or elevation of the feet as a result of head flexion.
- Increased flexion in the lower body as a result of head extension.
- Note any attempt to alter the hand position during testing (locking or rotation of the elbows) or arching and hollowing of the back. Arching and hollowing of the back may be an attempt to deflect the effect of the reflex in the arms but is not necessarily evidence of the reflex being present.
- Scoring for signs of the STNR in flexion and extension are listed in the following:

Scoring

Flexion

0. No response
1. Tremor in one or both arms in response to flexion of the head
2. Slight bending of the elbows
3. Definite bending of the arms as a result of head flexion and/or elevation of the feet
4. Bending of the arms to the floor

Extension

0. No response
1. Slight movement in the hips (flexion in the lower body)
2. Small movement in the hips
3. Definite movement in the hips
4. Movement of the bottom back onto the ankles so that the test subject is in the 'sitting cat' position

Tonic Labyrinthine Reflex (TLR): Erect test

In the infant, movement of the head through the mid-plane (flexion or extension of the head) will elicit changes in body position and muscle tonus.

When tested in infants and very young children, the test is usually carried out in a suspended supine position. However, as with the ATNR, as postural control and muscle tone develop, the reflex can be inhibited in positions where there is minimal challenge to balance and posture, as when lying supine, but fails to be inhibited as the demand on muscle tone required to maintain anti-gravity posture increases. An additional test for the TLR has been developed for use beyond the infancy period to assess the presence of the TLR in the erect position.

The patient is instructed to stand with feet together and arms by the sides with the eyes closed and to slowly tilt the head back 'as if looking towards the ceiling'. If the reflex is present in extension, either movement of the head as it passes *through* the mid-plane or when the head is in an extended position will result in a significant increase in extensor muscle tonus throughout the body.

(a)

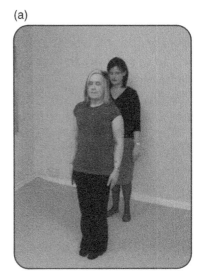

Figure 4.7a TLR test position.

The patient is then instructed to slowly bring the head forwards 'as if looking down at your toes'. If the reflex is present in flexion as the head is moved forwards through the mid-plane into flexion, there will be significant increase in flexor muscle tonus through the entire length of the body.

As distribution of muscle tone is involved in the control of both balance and posture, if the reflex is present in either position, head movement through the mid-plane can interfere with control of upright balance.

Traces of the tonic labyrinthine reflex can persist under different postural conditions up to 3½ years of age but should be suppressed from this time.

Test procedure

Test position: standing

Please note it is important for the tester to stand behind or beside the patient throughout the test procedure, as movement of the head can result in loss of balance:

(b)

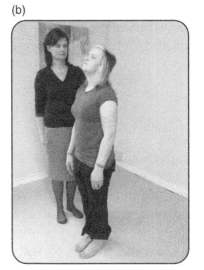

Figure 4.7b TLR with head extension.

- Instruct the subject to stand with feet together and arms straight at the sides of the body. Tester stands behind or beside the subject (Figure 4.7a, Figure 4.7b and Figure 4.7c).

(c)

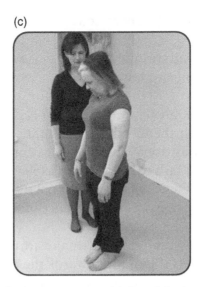

Figure 4.7c TLR with head flexion.

- Slowly tilt the head back into an extended position, *as if looking up at the ceiling*, and then instruct the subject to close the eyes. (Stand behind or beside to support in case of loss of balance and do not allow the patient to over-extend the head.)
- Pause for up to five seconds when the head is in the extended position.
- Slowly move the head forwards, *as if looking down at your toes*, and maintain that position for a further five seconds.
- Slowly move the head back into the extended position.
- Repeat the sequence three to four times.

Observations

- Note any loss of balance or alteration of balance in response to flexion or extension of the head or as the head moves through the mid-plane.
- Observe any compensatory changes in muscle tone at the back of the knees and gripping or extension in the toes which occurs when the head is moved through the mid-plane.
- Ask the patient how he/she feels immediately after testing, and note any comments about feelings of dizziness, nausea, disorientation or anxiety during the testing – which might indicate faulty vestibular–proprioceptive interaction and/or the residual presence of the tonic labyrinthine reflex.

Scoring

0. No response.
1. Slight alteration of balance or alteration in muscle tone, particularly in the lower half of the body as a result of change in head position.
2. Impairment of balance during test and/or alteration of muscle tone.
3. Near loss of balance and/or alteration of muscle tone and/or disorientation as a result of test procedure.
4. Loss of balance and/or marked adjustment in muscle tone in attempt to stabilize balance. This may be accompanied by dizziness, nausea, disorientation and/or anxiety.

Moro reflex

Standard test (adapted by Goddard Blythe for use with children and adults, 2003)

Test procedure

Test position

- Supine with a small cushion placed under the middle of the back at shoulder level
- Arms flexed and held up as if getting ready to clasp a large ball but with wrists flexed
- Head supported by the tester, slightly flexed and above the level of the spine
- Eyes closed as in Figure 4.8a

(a)

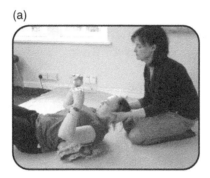

Figure 4.8a Test position for the adapted standard test for the Moro reflex.

Instruction

In a few moments time, I am going to let your head drop back a little way. I promise your head will not hit the floor. I want you to try to keep the rest of your body still in the test position.

- When the subject's head is relaxed, supported by the tester's hands, the tester drops the head at least 2 inches (5 cm) below the level of the spine, always keeping the hands beneath the subject's head so that the head is caught **before** it touches the floor (Figure 4.8b).

(b)

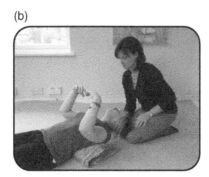

Figure 4.8b Head position *after* applying the test stimulus. No reflex present.

NB. *Both* hands should be used to support the head *during* the test procedure.

Observations

- Can the subject maintain the arm position when the head drops, or is there abduction of the arms?
- How much abduction of the arms do you observe?
- Is the subject visibly distressed by the procedure (over-arousal)?
- Is there a marked alteration in subject's colour following the procedure, that is, pallor or reddening of the skin?
- Is the subject very quiet or withdrawn following the test procedure?
- Is the subject unable to relax the neck muscles to allow the head to drop?

(c)

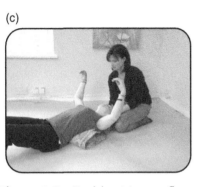

Figure 4.8c Positive Moro reflex following use of the adapted standard test.

Scoring

0. No movement of the arms and no sign of distress or discomfort
1. Fractional movement of the arms outwards (abduction) or momentary freeze
2. Definite arm involvement and slight freeze reaction and/or signs of emotional discomfort following test procedure
3. Partial abduction of the arms and dislike of test procedure
4. Abduction of the arms and/or visibly distressed by the test procedure (Figure 4.8c)

If the subject is unable to 'let go' for the head to drop, this *might* suggest the Moro reflex is present.

Erect (drag) test for the Moro reflex

An erect test for the Moro reflex was devised by two INPP practitioners when it became evident that the standard test used with neonates in the supine position did not always elicit an active Moro reflex in older individuals, particularly adults who have developed muscular resistance, 'body armouring'.[13]

In older children and adults, in whom either vestibular or postural problems are present, the Moro reflex may only be evident on the erect test, when there is increased gravitational challenge to the postural system. In these cases, the Moro reflex may not be elicited when tested in the supine position.† The erect test for the Moro reflex has since been adapted to make it easier to administer and is known as the erect (drag) test for the Moro reflex.

Test procedure

Test position

Erect, standing with feet together, arms bent, wrists relaxed, head extended and eyes closed as in Figure 4.8d.

Tester stands behind the subject ready to support the weight of the subject.

NB: Do *not* attempt this test with a subject who is taller or heavier than the tester.

(d)

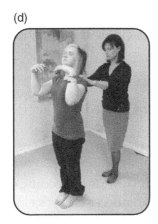

Figure 4.8d Test position for the erect 'drag back' test.

Instructions

- Assume testing position standing behind the subject (Figure 4.8d).
- Tester should stand with one foot in front of the other and hands placed on the shoulders ready to support the weight of the test subject. Instruct the subject:

Keeping your body straight, I want you lean back on to your heels like a pillar, allowing me to take your weight. I will let you drop a very small distance (approximately 10 degrees) and I promise I will catch you. Try to keep the remainder of your body in the test position if you can

---

†Retention of the Moro reflex may be secondary to underlying postural dysfunction, and when balance and posture improve, the Moro reflex recedes.

(e)

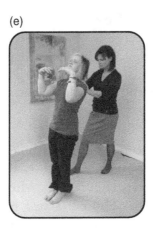

Figure 4.8e Lowered position for the erect 'drag back' test for the Moro reflex.

- With the patient's weight distributed on to their heels, leaning back supported by the tester, allow the patient to drop a distance of about 10° (Figure 4.8e).
- *Catch* the patient before they fall any further.
- Do *not* take patient beyond an angle of 30° before allowing them to drop. If the patient is anxious or very sensitive to vestibular stimulation, it may not be necessary to take them as far as 30° before allowing them to drop a short distance.
- You may also observe abduction in the arms when the patient is placed in the test position *before* allowing the patient to fall a short distance. If you observe this sign, it is not necessary to proceed further with the test.

Observations

- Can the subject maintain the arm position when falling back, or is there abduction of the arms?
- How much abduction of the arms do you observe?
- Is the subject visibly distressed by the procedure?
- Is there a marked alteration in subject's colour following the procedure, that is, pallor or reddening of the skin?
- Is the subject very quiet or withdrawn following the test procedure?
- Is the subject distressed by the test procedure (hyper-arousal)?
- Is the subject unwilling to lean back far enough to carry out the test or become extremely anxious when placed in the test position with the head extended and eyes closed? This may be indicative of a TLR and/or Moro reflex being present.
- Does the subject take a step instead of allowing him/herself to fall?

Scoring

0. No reaction and arms remain in testing position.
1. Minimal abduction of the arms.
2. Definite partial abduction of the arms and intake of breath.
3. Arms abducted by 75% and/or subject 'shaken' by test procedure.
4. Full abduction of the arms and/or subject distressed by test procedure.

4.7 Adult screening test

Score sheet

	1st assessment	2nd assessment
Date **Name** **Code number** **Age of subject**		
Romberg test (eyes open)	0 1 2 3 4	0 1 2 3 4
Romberg test (eyes closed)	0 1 2 3 4	0 1 2 3 4
Mann test (eyes open)	0 1 2 3 4	0 1 2 3 4
Mann test (eyes closed)	0 1 2 3 4	0 1 2 3 4
Tandem walk – forwards	0 1 2 3 4	0 1 2 3 4
Tandem walk – backwards	0 1 2 3 4	0 1 2 3 4
Fog walk – forwards	0 1 2 3 4	0 1 2 3 4
Fog walk – backwards	0 1 2 3 4	0 1 2 3 4
Asymmetrical tonic neck reflex quadruped test – right	0 1 2 3 4	0 1 2 3 4
Asymmetrical tonic neck reflex quadruped test – left	0 1 2 3 4	0 1 2 3 4
Asymmetrical Tonic Neck Reflex – adapted Hoff-Schilder test – right	0 1 2 3 4	0 1 2 3 4
Asymmetrical Tonic Neck Reflex – adapted Hoff-Schilder test – left	0 1 2 3 4	0 1 2 3 4
Symmetrical tonic neck reflex – flexion	0 1 2 3 4	0 1 2 3 4
Symmetrical tonic neck reflex – extension	0 1 2 3 4	0 1 2 3 4
Tonic labyrinthine reflex – flexion	0 1 2 3 4	0 1 2 3 4
Tonic labyrinthine reflex – extension	0 1 2 3 4	0 1 2 3 4
Moro reflex – supine (standard test)	0 1 2 3 4	0 1 2 3 4
Moro reflex – erect (drag back)	0 1 2 3 4	0 1 2 3 4
Total	**/72**	**/72**
Percentage score: total/72 x 100		

Observation sheet

1st assessment	*2nd assessment*
Date	
Name	
Code number	
Age of subject	
Romberg test (eyes open)	
Romberg test (eyes closed)	
Mann test (eyes open)	
Mann test (eyes closed)	
Tandem walk – forwards	
Tandem walk – backwards	
Fog walk – forwards	
Fog walk – backwards	
Asymmetrical tonic neck reflex quadruped test – right	
Asymmetrical tonic neck reflex quadruped test – left	
Asymmetrical Tonic Neck Reflex – adapted Hoff-Schilder test – right	
Asymmetrical Tonic Neck Reflex – adapted Hoff-Schilder test – left	
Symmetrical tonic neck reflex – flexion	
Symmetrical tonic neck reflex – extension	
Tonic labyrinthine reflex – flexion	
Tonic labyrinthine reflex – extension	
Moro reflex – supine	
Moro reflex – erect	

Additional score and observation sheets can be downloaded from http://www.inpp.org.uk/scoresheets

4.8 Interpreting the scores

Scores are interpreted in five categories:

1. No Abnormality Detected (NAD)
2. **Low** score < 25%
3. **Medium** score 25–49%
4. **High score** 50–74%
5. **Very high score** 75–100%

1	NAD	No action required
2	Low score	May benefit from INPP method
3	Medium score	INPP diagnostic assessment and individual programme indicated
4	High score	INPP diagnostic assessment and individual programme indicated
5	Very high score	Referral for further medical investigations indicated. (Following appropriate assessment, an INPP programme may also be of benefit) *Please note that in adults presenting with symptoms of anxiety, agoraphobia or panic disorder, it is recommended that independent counselling is made available to run concurrently with the programme if required*

When this screening test is used with adults presenting with agoraphobia with or without panic disorder or chronic acute anxiety states, if the patient displays disturbed emotional reaction to any of the vestibular tests, this might indicate that the aetiology of the 'symptoms' resides in vestibular dysfunction. The more extreme the emotional reaction (provided there is no previously confirmed pathology), the greater the probability that on further assessment vestibular dysfunction or neuromotor immaturity will be found to be playing a significant part in the presenting symptomatology.

Tests which indicate abnormal vestibular involvement in the presenting reaction are:

- Romberg test
- Hoff–Schilder test for the Asymmetrical Tonic Neck Reflex (ATNR)
- Erect test for the Tonic Labyrinthine Reflex (TLR)
- Standard test for the Moro reflex
- Erect test for the Moro reflex

If the tests for gross muscle coordination and balance elicit low scores but subsequent tests for the tonic labyrinthine reflex and Hoff–Schilder test for the asymmetrical tonic neck reflex elicit a strong positive reaction, this might indicate vestibular and/or postural involvement in the presenting symptoms, and accordingly, the patient should be referred to an INPP practitioner, qualified to work with adults for further assessment.

If there is a strong reaction to the test for the Moro reflex, this could be a significant underlying factor in panic disorder. Provided no pathology has been identified, this would be an indication for referral to an INPP practitioner.[‡]

[‡]See note †.

If a patient is unable to complete the Romberg test together with a fully retained ATNR, an additional test for the Babinski reflex should be carried out. If all three signs are abnormal, the patient should be referred for further neurological investigations.

References

1 Davies, R (2004) Bed-side neuro-otological examination and interpretation of commonly used investigations. *Journal of Neurology, Neurosurgery & Psychiatry*, **75**: iv32–iv44.

2 Griffiths, TD, Sigmundsson, T, Takei, N, Rowe, D and Murray, RM (1998) Neurological abnormalities in familial and sporadic schizophrenia. *Brain*, **121**: 191–203.

3 Heinrichs, DW and Buchanan, RW (1988) Significance and meaning of neurological signs in schizophrenia. *American Journal of Psychiatry*, **145**: 11–18.

4 Agrawal, Y, Carey, JP, Howard, J, Hoffman, HJ, Sklare, DA and Schubert, MC (2011) The modified Romberg balance test: normative data in U.S. adults. *Otology & Neurotology*, **32**: 1309–1311.

5 Beuret, LJ (2011) Personal communication.

6 Steffen, T (2012) Romberg (R) and Sharpened Romberg (SR). http://www.exercisepd.com/uploads/3/5/3/1/3531021/romberg.nov2012.pdf. Accessed January 17, 2014.

7 Perkowski, L, Stroup-Benham, C, Markides, K, Lichtenstein, M, Angel, R, Guralnik, J and Goodwin, JS (1998) Lower-extremity functioning in older Mexican Americans and its association with medical problems. *Journal of the American Geriatrics Society*, **46**(4), 411–418.

8 Seeman, T, Charpentier, P, Berkman, L, Tinetti, M, Guralnik, J, Albert, M, Blazer, D and Rowe, JW et al (1994) Predicting changes in physical performance in a high-functioning elderly cohort: MacArthur studies of successful aging. *Journal of Gerontology*, **49**(3): M97–M108.

9 Guralnik, JM, Simonsick, EM, Ferrucci, L, Glynn, RJ, Berkman, LF, Blazer, DG., Scherr, PA and Wallace, RB. (1994) A short physical performance battery assessing lower extremity function: association with self-reported disability and prediction of mortality and nursing home admission. *Journals of Gerontology*, **49**(2): M85–M94.

10 Fog, E and Fog, M (1963) Cerebral inhibition examined by associated movements. In: MacKeith, R and Bax, M (eds), *Minimal cerebral dysfunction. Papers from the international study group held at Oxford. September 1962*. William Heinemann Medical Books Ltd., London.

11 Ayres, AJ (1978) *Sensory integration and learning disorders*. Western Psychological Services, Los Angeles, CA.

12 Hoff, H and Schilder, P (1927) *Die Lagereflexe des Menschen. Klinische Untersuchungen über Haltungs- und Stellreflexe und verwandte Phänomene*. Julius Springer, Wien.

13 Bennett, R (1988) *The hidden Moro*. Private Publication.

Resources

Additional Observation and Score Sheets

Additional score and observation sheets may be downloaded from: http://www.inpp.org.uk/scoresheets

Training in The INPP Method

INPP provides training in the use of:

1. *Assessing Neuromotor Readiness for Learning. The INPP Developmental Screening Test and School Intervention Programme.*
   a. **One day course for teachers and educators**
2. *Neuromotor Immaturity in Children and Adults. The INPP Screening Test for Clinicians and Health Professionals.*
   b. **One day course for clinicians and health practitioners.**
3. Practitioner training course
   c. **Four module post-graduate course run over a nine month period.**

Further information about training in The INPP Method, research and publications can be found at: www.inpp.org.uk

Information about international courses approved by INPP can be found by following the contact details at: www.inpp.org.uk

Other Books by Sally Goddard Blythe*

Reflexes, Learning and Behavior, Fern Ridge Press, Eugene, OR, 2002.

The Well Balanced Child, Hawthorn Press, Stroud, 2005.

---

*Flyers are shown in the following pages.

What Babies and Children Really Need, Hawthorn Press, Stroud, 2008.

Attention, Balance and Coordination: The A,B,C of Learning Success, Wiley-Blackwell, Chichester, 2009.

The Genius of Natural Childhood, Hawthorn Press, Stroud, 2011.

Assessing Neuromotor Readiness for Learning. The INPP Developmental Screening Test and School Intervention Programme, Wiley-Blackwell, Chichester, 2012.

Books on The INPP Method

An Organic Basis for Neurosis and Educational Difficulties by Peter Blythe and David McGlown, Insight Publications, Chester.

Further information about the author can be found at: www.sallygoddardblythe.co.uk

Reflexes, Learning & Behavior

A Window into the Child's Mind

by Sally Goddard

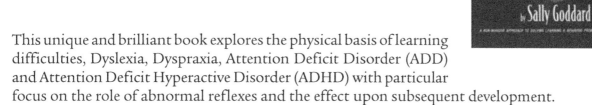

This unique and brilliant book explores the physical basis of learning difficulties, Dyslexia, Dyspraxia, Attention Deficit Disorder (ADD) and Attention Deficit Hyperactive Disorder (ADHD) with particular focus on the role of abnormal reflexes and the effect upon subsequent development.

Sally Goddard, Director of The Institute for Neuro-Physiological Psychology, Chester, explains how the reflexes of infancy (primitive and postural) can affect the learning ability of the child if they are not inhibited and integrated by the developing brain in the first three years of life. Each reflex is described together with its function in normal development, and its impact upon learning and behaviour if it remains active beyond the normal period.

Simple tests for the reflexes that are crucial to education are described, together with suggestions for suitable remedial intervention. A brief history of how current methods of intervention designed to correct abnormal reflexes have evolved is included and a summary of some of the relevant research in the field.

This book is essential reading for parents, teachers, psychologists, optometrists and anyone involved in the assessment, education and management of children and their problems. It explains *why* certain children are unable to benefit from the same teaching methods as their peers and why they remain immature in other aspects of their lives.

The Well Balanced Child

Movement and Early Learning

Sally Goddard Blythe

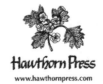 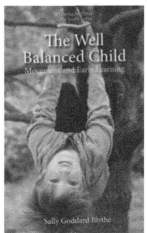

Concern about the increasingly sedentary lifestyle of young children is reaching unprecedented levels. Around a third of British children are overweight, reflecting the decline of traditional outdoor pursuits in favour of electronic games and television. A raft of studies shows that the early years are a crucial window of opportunity during which the brain is primed for learning through exercising the body and the senses. Yet children of today have less movement opportunities in their daily lives than any previous generation.

The Well Balanced Child is a passionate manifesto for the importance of movement in early years education. Author Sally Goddard Blythe, a leading expert in neuro-physiological development, argues for a 'whole body' approach to learning which integrates the brain, senses, movement, music and play. Using case studies and the latest research, she demonstrates:

- Why movement matters
- How music helps brain development
- The role of nutrition, the brain and child growth
- Practical tips for parents and educators to help children with learning and behavioural problems

Sally Goddard Blythe is Director of the Institute for Neuro-Physiological Psychology (INPP) in Chester, which researches the effects of neurological dysfunction in specific learning difficulties and devises effective learning programmes. She researches, consults and advises schools, parents and professionals.

What Babies and Children Really Need

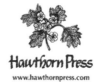

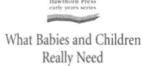

Sally Goddard Blythe

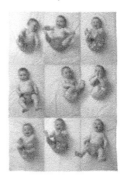

How mothers and fathers can nurture children's growth for health and wellbeing.

This book represents a milestone in our understanding of child development and what parents can do to provide their children with the best start in life. *What Babies and Children Really Need* examines the crucial early years from a *child's* perspective and concludes that changes in society over the past 50 years have unleashed a crisis in childhood.

Author Sally Goddard Blythe draws on the latest scientific research and clinical practice to demonstrate how a baby's relationship with its mother has a lasting and fundamental impact. She argues that trends such as delayed motherhood, limited uptake of breastfeeding and early return to work – driven by economic, social and political pressures – are undermining the key developmental milestones essential to success and wellbeing in later life. 'We need a state', says Goddard Blythe, 'that gives children their parents, and most of all, gives babies their mothers back'.

What Babies and Children Really Need concludes with a rallying cry for a new Charter for Childhood founded on the four main pillars of child development: nutrition – the biochemical basis for life; affection, nurture and engagement; stimulating sensory experience and motor skills through physical play; and discipline in its true sense meaning 'instruction, correction, training in action and control'.

Outline of contents

1. Conception and society – the politics of fertility
2. Does early development matter?
3. Events surrounding birth
4. Events following birth – risk factors
5. Breastfeeding
6. Movement instinct
7. Language instinct
8. Building on the first year – the neuroscience of developing emotions
9. Factors parents can control
10. What needs to be done?

Sally Goddard Blythe is Director of the Institute for Neuro-Physiological Psychology in Chester which researches the effects of neurological dysfunction in specific learning difficulties and devises effective remedial programmes. Her other books include *The Well Balanced Child* (also published by Hawthorn Press), 978-1-903458-76-1, £16.99 216 × 138 mm, 368 pp. Published May 2008.

Early Years series

Hawthorn Press, 1 Lansdown Lane, Lansdown Stroud GL5 1BJ, Tel: +44 (0) 1453 757040, Fax: +44 (0) 1453 751138, Email: sales@hawthornpress.

Attention, Balance and Coordination
The A.B.C. of Learning Success
Sally Goddard Blythe

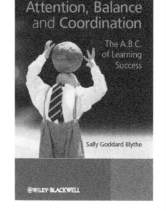

In *Attention, Balance and Coordination*, Sally Goddard Blythe explores the physical basis for learning. She explains the importance of early reflexes, their functions in early development and their effects on learning and behaviour if retained. Goddard Blythe also investigates the possible effects that these early reflexes have on other aspects of development such as posture, balance, motor skills and susceptibility to stress and anxiety in later life.

Attention, Balance and Coordination also includes:

- a review of relevant literature in the field
- a review of the origins of The Vestibular-Cerebellar Theory
- The Institute for Neuro-Physiological Psychology (INPP) Developmental Screening Questionnaire, together with an explanation on how its use and interpretation
- a chapter by Dr Peter Blythe looking at the development of the INPP Method
- effects of neuro-developmental delay in adolescents and adults

Attention, Balance and Coordination is the most up-to-date handbook for professionals involved in education and child development, providing a new understanding of the source of specific behavioural problems and educational under-achievement.

Sally Goddard Blythe is Director for the Institute of Neuro-Physiological Psychology in Chester, which specialises in the assessment and supervision of remediation programmes for children and adults with specific learning difficulties, agoraphobia and panic disorder. She is the author of a number of widely acclaimed books, including *Reflexes, Learning and Behaviour* (2002), *The Well-Balanced Child* (2005) and *What Babies and Children Really Need* (2008).

The Genius of Natural Childhood

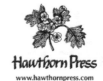

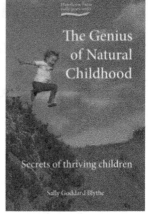

Secrets of thriving children

Sally Goddard Blythe

Many children are just not ready for school at age five. One reason may be that busy families have abandoned nursery rhymes, bedtime stories, singing lullabies and playing with their children. Sally Goddard Blythe uses neuroscience to show just why such 'old fashioned ways' are the secrets of thriving children in her eagerly awaited new book, *The Genius of Natural Childhood*.

Sally Goddard Blythe, director of The Institute for Neuro-Physiological Psychology, says that what is important is using music, singing and lullabies to playfully get a baby ready for language. She suggests using fairy tales to teach moral behaviour and empathy. She shows, using neuroscience, how movement with singing games such as *Pata-cake, Pat-a-cake* and rough and tumble play enable children to learn motor skills and self-control naturally.

Without such activities, a large proportion of five year olds are held back by baby reflexes, which can stop them holding a pencil properly or learning to read, for example. A Northern Ireland study found traces of baby reflexes in 48% of first year children and 35% of fourth years.

She says, 'It's alarming the proportion of children with immature motor skills when they start school, regardless of intelligence. A significant percentage of children have problems they don't need to have.

They seem to have missed out on early stages of development'.

Here are the secrets of thriving children – why early movement matters and how games develop children's motor skills. Sally Goddard Blythe offers a handy starter kit of stories, action games, songs and rhymes and explains:

- Why movement is essential for healthy brain development
- Just how music, songs, lullabies and nursery rhymes prepare the brain for language
- The importance of 'rough and tumble' play for emotional and social development
- How fairy tales help children face fears, develop empathy and moral behaviour
- The links between learning problems, sedentary lifestyles and over exposure to the electronic media
- What to look for if your child doesn't seem ready for school
- Favourite baby massage rhymes, action songs, finger plays and rhymes with Jane Williams of Gymbaroo

An inspiration for supporting young children – her engaging use of the latest neuroscientific insights show just why the 'old fashioned ways' often had it right all along. Dr Richard House, Roehampton University.

Sally Goddard Blythe's delightfully illustrated book is about the natural vitality of young children and how they can thrive'. Professor Colwyn Trevarthen, Child Psychology, The University of Edinburgh.

Sally Goddard Blythe is Director of the Institute for Neuro-Physiological Psychology in Chester, a research, training and clinical organisation which has pioneered research into the neuroscience of specific learning difficulties. An international authority on remedial programmes, she has authored numerous professional papers and books such as *Reflexes, Learning and Behaviour, Attention Balance and Coordination: The A.B.C. of Learning Success, What Babies and Children Really Need* and *The Well Balanced Child* – now widely translated. She is also the author of a screening test and movement programme for schools due to be published later this year. *The Genius of Natural Childhood* is published by Hawthorn Press in the Early Years' Series, price £14.99.

June 2011, ISBN: 978-1-907359-04-0, Paperback 234 × 156 mm, 240 pp.

Assessing Neuromotor Readiness for Learning

The INPP developmental screening test and school intervention programme

Sally Goddard Blythe

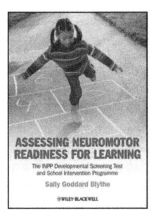

Assessing Neuromotor Readiness for Learning is a substantially revised and expanded edition of a long established INPP training manual that has been consistently proven in practice.

- It includes tests for children, a developmental movement programme and online access to INPP video training materials.
- It is based on the proven INPP model for neuro-motor development screening and intervention, which is unique in having been rigorously evaluated in research and practice.
- It expands and revises an INPP manual which has previously only been available to training customers, and which is a foundation stone of the overall INPP approach.
- It places emphasis on assessing children's physical development and how neuro-motor skills provide the foundations for learning success.
- It includes batteries of tests for younger and older children, a developmental movement programme and online access to INPP video training materials.

Published 2012. Wiley-Blackwell.

Index

Neuromotor Immaturity in Children and Adults: The INPP Screening Test for Clinicians and Health Practitioners, First Edition. Sally Goddard Blythe.
© 2014 John Wiley & Sons, Ltd. Published 2014 by John Wiley & Sons, Ltd.